Weight
Loss
from
the
Inside Out

WEIGHT LOSS from the INSIDE OUT

Help for the Compulsive Eater

MARION BILICH

The Seabury Press • New York

1983
The Seabury Press
815 Second Avenue
New York, N.Y. 10017

Copyright © 1983 by Marion Bilich

All rights reserved. No part of this book may be reproduced, stored in a retrieval system, or transmitted, in any form or by any means, electronic, mechanical, photocopying, recording, or otherwise, without the written permission of The Seabury Press.

Printed in the United States of America.

Library of Congress Cataloging in Publication Data

Bilich, Marion.
Weight loss from the inside out.

Bibliography: p. 191
Includes index.
1. Reducing diets.   2. Reducing—Psychological aspects.   3. Obesity—Psychological aspects.   4. Compulsive behavior.   I. Title.
RM222.2.B54   1983   613.2'5'019   83-633
ISBN 0-8164-2485-3

To Susie Orbach,
with all my love,
for her teaching
and support

Contents

Preface ix

Introduction 1

one • My Journey: Bulimia   7

two • The Power of Fat   28

three • The Reality of Thin   58

four • Bodywork   81

five • Eating Awareness   111

six • The Power of Food   144

seven • Putting It All Together and Losing Weight   160

A Note to Psychotherapists   179

Notes   188

Suggested Reading   191

Index   193

Acknowledgments

I would like to thank my husband, Chuck, and my daughter, Karin, for their much-appreciated support while I was writing this book. Thanks also to Sylvia Yellin Pierce, my mother, and to Ronnie Yellin Charme, my sister, and to Pearl and Sonny Posin for their love and support.

Muriel Belsky and Jeff Lawrence were two people who helped me keep going when I hit snags in my writing. I would also like to thank the others who contributed to this book with their ideas and enthusiastic support: Carol Cohen, Mimi Coon, Loretta Barbetti, Nancy Kahn, Madelyn Larsen, Paula Marcisak, Judy Spindel, and Judy and Howard Steinberg. Special thanks to my patients, who taught me so much and who provided me with many of the ideas for this book.

Preface

"An inner journey"—the words struck me immediately. Eda Leshan was being interviewed on television about her latest book, *Winning the Losing Battle*, and she had just referred to her period of weight reduction as an inner journey. That short phrase expressed the essence of my own views both personally and professionally, and at that moment the idea for my own book was conceived.

Losing weight is relatively simple, but getting over a compulsive eating problem and keeping the excess weight off permanently requires much more than a diet. It requires a journey inside one's mind, a trip which aims at discovering unconscious motivations and even hidden fears. It can be a long and difficult journey and therefore few of us ever take it. Perhaps that is who so few women keep their weight off permanently.

I undertook such an inner journey some years ago, and as a therapist have helped many others to do so. This book is about our experiences, but more importantly it will guide you through your own inner journey.

Introduction

Two questions may come immediately to mind: "Why another diet book?" and "Why a guide for women?"

To begin with, this is *not* a diet book—quite the contrary, since dieting, as we shall see, is not a means to permanent weight loss. True, when the time comes to lose weight, some of my clients do choose to diet. However, the key phrase here is "when the time comes to lose weight," because for most compulsive eaters permanent weight loss can only come after much psychological preparation. It is the thesis of this book that for women with compulsive eating problems, overweight is not simply the result of overindulgence, lack of will power, or even bad eating habits. Fat and the compulsive eating problem itself are performing functions in a woman's life, and to lose weight without identifying these functions can only lead to failure.

There are many kinds of diet books. Some present fantastic new diets which enable the dieter to shed pounds quickly. These diets, though often unhealthy, do work, but in the long run lost weight is regained.[1] There are also diet books which aim at modifying behavior, correcting bad habits, or arranging an environment that discourages overeating. Such books have some merit because compulsive eaters tend to eat in response to external factors: for example, the sight or smell of food, or a social situation that calls for eating. Unfortunately, these behavioral approaches deal with only one aspect of the problem and therefore can offer only partial success. Still other books focus on the use of self-hypnosis to control weight. Based on my experiences, both personally and professionally, self-hypnosis techniques work well *only if the person applying them has no stake in maintaining her problem.*[2] A great drawback to using diet books is that, for the most part, they do not take into account the unconscious needs many women have to maintain their fat and compulsive eating behavior.

I have an even greater reservation about the helpfulness of diets—a reservation which stems from the way women in particular have been taught to think about themselves. Women have long been encouraged not to trust their body signals, but to rely instead on some outside, presumably more knowledgeable authority, to determine their physical needs. Diets are merely another such prescription from authorities (usually men), who inform the woman what, when, where, and how much to eat. It is the aim of this book to help women discover more about their bodily needs, especially those centering upon food and eating, and to help them develop new ways of eating which are consistent with their needs.

Clearly you are not about to read "just another diet book." But what about the second question posed earlier: "Why a guide for women?" "Don't men get fat?" you may ask. "Aren't men out of touch with their body signals too?" To these questions I must answer "yes," with reservations. Men overeat. Men use food to meet emotional needs. They eat when they are bored, frustrated, or depressed—just like women. Their fat may even be serving a function in their lives. One man I know is aware that he got fat because he is short and does not feel masculine. To him, being fat means being big and manly. Yet despite the similarities, there are differences which make the compulsive eating problem not only more prevalent among women, but more far-reaching in its consequences.

In our culture, men are judged by their jobs and how much money they make—a situation which creates its own problems—but while a fat man may be discriminated against in the job market, his professional abilities and assets usually count for far more. Women, on the other hand, have tended to be judged primarily by their physical appearance. There is an ideal female body to which most women aspire. Though it is not clear just what constitutes this perfect body, it *is* clear that its dimensions change periodically. In the past two decades this standard has increasingly emphasized slimness ("You can never be too rich or too thin"). Along with the ideal body are supposed to come a man, social position, money, and even happiness. The constant cycle of dieting and subsequent weight gain stems in part from the never ending battle to meet an unrealistic standard, to attain the perfect body and all the things that go with it. For some women, getting fat is a way of dropping out of the rat race. "I'll never have a great figure, even if I do get thin," many of my clients have said, "so why keep trying?" Other women view their fat as a statement of rebellion: "I refuse to be that ideal Playmate men want me to be." (It is important to point out that most often these feelings are unconscious.)

Another aspect of women's experience which often manifests itself in compulsive eating is related to the nurturing role for which most women have been trained. Having been encouraged, even expected to care for husband, children, friends, relatives, even strangers, few women have learned how to care for or nurture themselves. The needs of others always come first. In many cases the only thing a woman may give herself is food; the only time she may allow for herself is time to eat. Similarly, she may not have learned—and certainly was not encouraged—to set limits, to say "no." Fat becomes a way of saying "no" to the world—"No, I won't be what you want. No, I won't do what you want. I can't. See, I'm too fat." Overeating, as well, can be a means of expressing rebellion.

It is not my intent to turn my patients into selfish women who care only for themselves. On the contrary, sometimes the needs of others do come first, but it is imperative that a woman experience some control in her life, that she weigh her needs against another's, that she herself decide whose needs will be met first. So often in the attempt to deny these basic human drives, women pretend they have no needs, and if women are out of touch with their emotional needs, it is not surprising that they would be out of touch with their physical needs as well, including those concerning food.

The experience of Jean, a patient in one of my groups, illustrates this point. Jean had been making much progress both in group and private therapy. As she allowed herself to become aware of new thoughts, feelings, and desires, her awareness of her food needs also sharpened. She began to eat less and began losing weight. She was amazed at each new discovery, however small; for instance, the realization that it was not the food that made restaurant dining so attractive, but the atmosphere, the social contact, the time to relax. As she began to realize what made her happy, her focus shifted from food to these other areas. However, when circumstances in her life changed, so did her ability to attend to her needs. In fact, due to a life crisis which affected all the members of her family, Jean felt she had to subordinate her needs to those of her young children and husband. She was under tremendous pressure but refused to share her fears and weariness with others.

It was about this time that she came to her group session complaining that she was gaining weight and saying that perhaps she should quit the group. The other women, aware of the crisis in Jean's life, urged her to stay on and helped her explore what was happening with her eating. Suddenly, she broke down and cried, "I can't even let myself cry at home. If I do, my feelings will come out and my family will know I'm not so strong." It was clear that Jean had not been allowing herself to have needs of her own, and shutting off the feelings meant being out of touch with *all* needs, physical as well as emotional; hence, the compulsive eating. Even the program of physical exercise which she had begun months before as an outlet for anger and tension had been discontinued, as she shut off all contact with her own needs and desires.

The connection between fat and the position of women in our society is an even more complex issue than I have presented here,[3] but these examples illustrate why I have chosen to write this guide primarily for women. There is another reason I have written this book for women, and it stems from the kinship and love I feel for my sex. Each patient who comes to me for help is being hampered in her full development by a problem which results in many ways from the position women have long held in our culture. Though initially most women come to my groups to lose weight, as the therapy develops the weight loss often becomes secondary, and these women begin to tackle issues in their lives which were previously hidden by their preoccupation with fat and eating. As the focus shifts, for example, from "I'm too fat" to "I need to learn to express anger instead of eating it away," a woman begins to blossom. A compulsive eating problem, and all the thinking and worrying and planning that goes with it, keeps a woman from developing fully. As long as fat and overeating are seen as a sickness, or as a symptom of underlying emotional problems, women will continue to be mistreated by the helping professions. Viewing fat in women in its social context, as a response and adaptation to difficult social circumstances, gives one a perspective that leads to a more effective approach to the problem.

Many of the ideas presented in this book are going to shake you up. In fact, you may initially view them with disbelief. I am going to tell you that no matter how much you consciously desire to lose weight there are *unconscious* needs and motivations that have prevented you from doing so. I am going to discuss your fears about getting thin. Your initial reaction is likely to be, "How could this ugly fat be doing anything but harm, and what could possibly be scary about being thin? I was thin before, and it wasn't scary." To this I ask, "Then why did you regain all the weight?" Perhaps then you might start to question, "Why *did* I gain the weight back?" Once you begin to think in these terms, you are on your way. The inner journey has begun.

I do not ask you to suspend judgment and swallow whole the ideas presented here, but I do ask that you keep an open mind and at least give them consideration. It is important, though, to realize that no single book or person has all the answers for you. You must take from this book what you can and apply it in your own way. If you are currently on a successful diet, the eating approach presented in Chapter 5 may not appeal to you, but there may be much to gain from the exploration of the realities and unrealistic expectations associated with being thin. You may find little in common with my patients who have used their fat as a means of protection; yet you may learn much from the section on the "power" of food. Each woman will have her own unique needs and her own inner journey. This book can be her guide.

one

My Journey: Bulimia

My own journey began in the early 1970s and led me through many twists and turns to a profession aimed at helping other women overcome their eating disorders. My eating problem, though it had no name in those days and was generally unknown to both the public and psychotherapists alike, was bulimia. Bulimia, bulimarexia, the binge-purge syndrome—all these terms describe an eating disorder which has gained much prominence in recent years. It is now estimated that 15 to 20 percent of all college women are afflicted with this disorder to some extent. Newspaper articles and television shows devoted to the topic abound, and on one segment of a popular news program even Jane Fonda surprised many with her confession that she, too, was once bulimic.

What is bulimia? It is an eating disorder that afflicts primarily young, upper- and middle-class females. The typical eating pattern of a bulimic consists of huge binges, followed by attempts to purge oneself of the food. A typical binge might consist of a box of cookies, a half gallon of ice cream, a bag of potato chips and a frozen cheese cake. The calorie count of a binge can range from 2,000 up to 55,000 calories at one sitting. Yet the average bulimic manages to maintain her weight within normal standards. In fact, most bulimic women appear thin. They maintain these low weights through the purges that follow each binge. A purge might consist of one or more of the following: laxatives, diuretics, emetics or self-induced vomiting, diet pills, stringent dieting or fasts, and excessive exercise. A woman with bulimia never eats "normally." She is either dieting strenuously ("under control"), binging, or purging. My own experience with bulimia will perhaps help to clarify this increasingly common, but still mystifying disorder.

I had always been slightly chubby as an adolescent, but never to the point where people would have labeled me as fat. My father, however, was fat and feared that I would end up like him. Then at eighteen years of age, prompted by a comment from my boyfriend that I was getting a little heavy, I embarked on my first diet, cutting out lunches and eating sparse dinners. Within four months I had lost twenty pounds and was quite thin. I remember feeling good about my new thin body, and proud of my accomplishment. There had been no sense of deprivation or compulsiveness when I was on the diet, and the months that followed the weight loss were pleasant ones in which the lost weight was easily maintained.

Then, after a long illness, my father died on my first day of college. Two incidents stand out from the period immediately following his death. I remember looking in the mirror the day of the funeral, catching myself admiring my figure and how lovely I looked in my dress. Then, realizing what I was getting dressed *for*, I immediately felt pangs of guilt. "How could I be admiring myself, finding pleasure in my body, on the day of my father's funeral?" I thought. That night, I threw the dress away.

The second incident occurred the following day. I was walking down the stairs and, suddenly, thoughts of what I was going to eat came to mind. The thoughts continued throughout the day. This was the first time I had ever obsessed about food. By day's end, I had experienced my first binge, having eaten everything I could find in the house. Thus began my eating problem.

Though I realize the roots of that problem stem back to early childhood, it was after my father's death that the problem emerged. Increasingly, diets and binges became a regular part of my day. I became obsessed with thoughts of food and with a desire, a passion, to remain thin. Yet, the binges were increasing and even the strict 500-calorie-a-day diets to which I adhered when not on a binge were not enough to keep the weight from piling on. Somehow, I do not remember how or when, I discovered that if I were to vomit, the calories consumed on a binge would not be absorbed by my body. I began sticking my fingers down my throat once or twice a week, but within a few months, the forced vomiting had increased to several times a day. I felt no one else in the world was doing what I was doing and that certainly no one could understand. Though I talked constantly about diets and weight, I told no one about my vomiting, mentioned to no one the feelings of revulsion and self-disgust I experienced when picking out people's leftover food from the top of the garbage pail.

During this period I became increasingly depressed and isolated from my friends, and though I did well academically in college, I did little else. My life became organized around food—when I would eat, what, how much. Either I was planning out my 500-calorie diet or I was binging and purging. Food and dieting were never far from my mind, even during sleep. I was obsessed with thinness and had a morbid fear of getting fatter. Though by most standards I was never overweight, in my mind I was much too fat and therefore unacceptable.

To me, to be thin was the end-all, the ultimate achievement in life. Thin women seemed happy, together, relaxed, energetic, sexy, feminine. I wanted all those qualities for myself, never stopping to think that my view of what being thin was all about was a fantasy. No wonder I could not get as thin as I wanted. I was looking for a cureall, a panacea for all my problems, and I believed I would find salvation merely by losing a few pounds. I do not mean to imply that I was to *blame* for my fantasy about what life would be like as a thin woman. I was, as are women today, living in a culture which promoted this fantasy. I was taught by the media, by everything around me, that being thin and attractive was a major, if not the ultimate, goal in a young woman's life. I learned from commercials, from movies, from television that thin meant happy, energetic, sexy. While as an individual I could do little to change our society's treatment of women, I needed to learn that I could change my *response* to society's expectations of me. I could give up its myth that being thin was wonderful and the ultimate goal of a woman's life—but it was years before I reached that point.

Meanwhile I remained totally involved in my pursuit of thinness. No one knew the extent of my eating problem, other than that I was constantly dieting. When I married, my husband remained unaware of my binging and purging, though he realized that I had a serious problem with food. Despite my constant complaints about my weight and my constant attempts to draw him into my problem, he remained apart from it, realizing that his involvement could not help me.

I remember grocery shopping with him and often adding a cake to the shopping cart, explaining that I was buying the cake for him. Then, while he was away at class, I would eat half or three-quarters of the cake. I would run out to the store and replace the cake, so that he would not know what I had done. Yet he really did not care if I ate the cake or not. It did not matter to him what I ate. He never told me what I "should" or "shouldn't" do. Sometimes I tried to provoke him into judging me, telling him about all I had eaten while he was away (though the vomiting still remained my secret)—but he did not take the bait.

Fortunately, I had chosen as a partner a man who had the good sense not to become involved in my eating problem. His confidence in himself and his sense of self-worth allowed him to view me as a competent, intelligent woman and to foster my growth both intellectually and emotionally. Had he been a man of less sensitivity and sense of self, he might have encouraged my dependence on him and surely would have hindered my efforts to get over my eating problem. As a therapist, I have since seen many cases where this is so.

Over the years I tried many diets and diet programs. Only one, Overeaters Anonymous (O.A.), a self-help group patterned after Alcoholics Anonymous, provided any relief. More importantly, however, my experience in O.A. was the first step in my journey, since it taught me to focus on the psychological basis of my eating problem. Though I strongly disagree with some of the concepts of the O.A. program, particularly the view that compulsive eating is an illness, it provided me, as it does so many others, with a life line to help. There were several things I learned in O.A. which were of great help. Most important was the concept of taking one day—even one hour—at a time. Compulsive eaters tend to look back at their past behavior and feel guilty or hopeless about ever changing. They tend to look forward to tomorrow and worry. In my case, the hopelessness and guilt over yesterday and the fear and worry about tomorrow led to many large binges. From O.A. I learned to focus on myself in the "now," and this focus led to such questions as, "Am I hungry *now*?" — "What do I want to eat *now*?" — "What am I needing *now*?" This focus on the present became an integral part of my life and forms the basis of my work.

Another positive aspect of O.A. was the concept of calling on another for help when one is overeating. Like many compulsive eaters, I was unable to ask others for help, and certainly unable to stop a binge on my own. Through O.A. I learned that it was okay to depend on the help of another when I was not able to "go it alone." Once in a while I was able to interupt a binge long enough to call an O.A. friend (a sponsor) and, with her help, examine the feelings and needs underlying the binge.

My experience in O.A. was only a temporary solution, however. I always had difficulty accepting their notion that I had an incurable illness. I wanted to believe that some day I would be able to eat "normally." I tired of planning my O.A. diets and confessing to my sponsor when I had cheated. Overeaters Anonymous had launched me on my journey to overcoming bulimia, but now I was ready to move on.

Then, about nine years ago, I heard about two women who had developed a new approach to compulsive eating problems viewed from a feminist perspective. A few months later, I heard them on WBAI, a public radio station in New York, discussing their own experiences and those of their patients. What they had to say shook me up, but these two, Carol Munter and Susie Orbach, were soon to become my therapists and my guides on an inner journey that would last many years. The actual therapy group in which I participated lasted only six months, but during that time the groundwork was laid. While I was not completely over my eating problem by the time the group was terminated, I had gained tools and insights with which to continue my inner journey — and more, I no longer experienced the huge binges, no longer dieted, and no longer made food and fat the focus of my life. Though I continued to eat at times for emotional reasons, food no longer frightened me, and a half gallon of ice cream could sit untouched in the freezer for weeks. The vomiting had ceased almost entirely. Then, while I was in graduate school several months later, I began training with Susie Orbach.

What happened in those six months of group therapy to bring about so radical a change? The work I did during those months, as well as that which I developed over the years, is presented in this book. Each chapter will deal with one aspect of the problem, presenting new ideas and ways to implement them, as well as providing you with the experiences of both my patients and myself as we worked through our eating problems.

It is generally the belief of both therapists and patients that one cannot "get over" an eating disorder (especially bulimia or anorexia), but can merely gain control over the problem. It has been my experience and that of my patients that a woman can, indeed, after much work and soul-searching, free herself completely and forever of an eating problem. I am no longer bulimic. There is no issue of control involved. I no longer use food and fat and fantasies about being thin as ways of dealing with emotional problems in my life. The problems still remain. In fact, some of the same issues which plagued me during my bulimic years are still with me today. The difference is that I *deal* with them differently—food and fat are not tied up with them anymore. One really can get over an eating problem and be freed of it forever.

Let us look more closely at the problem of bulimia and how it is treated. As I stated in the beginning of the chapter, it is sometimes referred to as the binge-purge syndrome, since the bulimic will generally binge on huge quantities of food, then clear that food out of her body, chiefly through the use of laxatives, diuretics, and self-induced vomiting, before the food has had time to be digested. It is an insidious problem, beginning usually during the teen years, with an occasional binge and purge, but slowly the frequency of binges and subsequent purges increases, until they come several times a day. More and more time and energy become tied up in eating—planning diets, planning binges, eating, purging. Eventually, a woman finds herself spending days at a time doing little else than eating and vomiting. For most women, it gets harder and harder to vomit as time goes by, because the gag reflex is not as strong after weeks and months of constant vomiting.

Therefore the binges have to get larger. The more food you have in your stomach the easier it is to throw up. Women learn quickly that certain foods are easier to throw up than others, and that liquids often are necessary. The food eaten on a binge is no longer tasted, no longer enjoyed, but seems to serve only to stuff the stomach to the point where vomiting can occur. There are real reasons, emotional and physical, why these binges and purges occur with such frequency. As we will discuss later in this chapter, there is a reason for this eating behavior, as self-destructive as it may appear on the surface.

In one of the few studies on bulimia conducted in the 1970s, Marlene Boskind-Lohahl and Joyce Sirlin were able to identify certain characteristics common to most women who became bulimic. They selected 100 women who had responded to a college newspaper ad. The women ranged in age from eighteen to thirty and in general came from affluent, well educated families. Typically, they described their mothers as demanding, their fathers as distant, involved in their work. They seemed to have a greater than normal dependence on others' opinions of them in forming a sense of self-worth, especially the opinons of men. Most strongly characteristic was their fear of sexual rejection, and a belief that their acceptance was based primarily on appearance.[1]

Bulimic women also tend to have been "good girls." They usually appear thin, well-dressed, and attractive—certainly not the type of person one would expect to be suffering from an eating disorder. Older bulimic women may be very successful and accomplished—writers, dancers, artists, business executives, doctors—but despite high achievements, they tend to be low in self-esteem. It has also been found that bulimic women tend to have higher than average anxiety levels and show a higher frequency of clinical depression.

Bulimic women display an array of physical disorders, among them hypokalemia (low potassium levels) which can lead to death; infections of the salivary glands; tooth decay caused by stomach acids in the vomit; rupture of the esophagus and an imbalance of electrolytes, both of which, while rare, can lead to cardiac arrest (electrolytes are substances which conduct electrical impulses from one part of the body to another); kidney and liver damage, constipation, spastic colon, ulcers. While few women actually die from this potentially fatal disorder, the less serious complications such as tooth decay and intestinal disturbances are extremely common.

The origins of bulimia are largely unknown. What is known is that in addition to the personality characteristics listed above, there are certain life experiences that often precede the development of the disorder. In a study of thirty-four bulimic women conducted at the University of Minnesota Hospital it was discovered that the binge-purge syndrome almost always began after the completion of a sucessful diet coupled with a traumatic event, such as a loss of or separation from someone close to the woman. The median age for the onset of the disorder was eighteen. Most of the women in the study came from large families with a high incidence of alcoholism, weight problems, and depression.[2] (The parallels to my own experience startled me when I learned of this study. In my own case, the bulimic eating patterns developed at the age of eighteen, after a successful diet and the loss of my father. Though I did not come from a large family, there was a history of weight problems in my family. My father's problem with overweight and overeating contributed in some way to his death.)

These patterns, common to so many women who develop bulimia, though they do not explain why the syndrome develops, may help researchers to identify the causes of bulimia. Some researchers have found evidence of physiological causes of the disturbed eating patterns: electrical disturbances in the brain, similar to those of epilepsy, have been proposed as a cause in certain rare cases. According to David Rudnick, a psychiatrist who established UCLA's eating disorders clinic, this electrical brain disturbance can be suspected: "if binges are not premeditated; if there is an altered state of consciousness—confused, dreamy, trancelike—during or after the binge; or if there are strange bodily sensations or psychological flashes (jamais vû, déjà vû, hallucinations) followed by binging."[3] If the symptoms you have experienced are similar to those above, it will be necessary to see a doctor who can administer an EEG (electroencephalogram) to test the electrical patterns of your brain. Medication may be prescribed in such cases.

Though in most instances disturbed body functioning will not be the cause of the disorder, a physical explanation for bulimia has been proposed which would explain its increasing frequency in Western culture. As I have indicated, the aesthetic standards for acceptable body weights have become lower and lower in recent years. Women, even young girls, are encouraged to lower their weight through diet or by whatever means necessary to conform to this unrealistic standard; yet not every woman was meant to be so thin, and in attempting to lower their weight to levels lower than their bodies require to function, some women may actually be battling with their bodies. The body, malnourished and starving, needs the extra fat and food, and so increases the appetite. The woman may fight this increased appetite for a time, but eventually, especially when she is under stress, she breaks down, "gives in" to her appetite and binges. Then, in order to assure herself that no weight gain will occur she vomits the food and takes a laxative, which further increases her body's need for food, and so the cycle continues.

According to Susan Wooley of the University of Cincinnati Medical Center, "One hundred percent of the people want to be in the bottom 10 percent of a bell-shaped curve of normal weight distribution. This is especially true for women, many of whom try to maintain a weight that is below their normal set point."[4] Studies on starvation show that when people of normal weight lose a significant amount of weight, they start going on binges as soon as they have access to unlimited quantities of food. Wooley suggests "that the binges get worse with time because the repeated purges impede the body's ability to detect satiation; this results in a need for ever greater quantities of food to appease 'hunger.' "[5] As hard as it may seem at first, the only way out of this pattern is for the woman to find the weight level at which her body best functions, even if this means *gaining* weight. Such a step usually requires some psychotherapy in preparation and support. Though it is hard to entertain the idea of having to gain some weight, in some cases the bulimic behavior disappears once the patient has been able to maintain a slightly higher weight.

For most bulimics, the need to be extremely thin is related to how they view themselves. As we have seen, bulimic women tend to be more dependent than most on the opinions of others, especially men, in forming their sense of self-worth, and they view their worth as consisting primarily of their sexual attractiveness to men. Many of my patients have expressed the feeling that if a man does not find them attractive they feel worthless. One woman realized that as a child she had learned that by being attractive she was able to get attention and love. In fact, all she had been praised for as a child was her beauty. Despite her accomplishments (she was a highly successful physician) she still felt, "If I lost my beauty, there would be nothing left of me." Others have expressed the fear that if they got fat (which might mean gaining only five pounds), they would be unloved. Given such low self-esteem and the degree to which any sense of self worth they do feel is tied into men's reactions to their physical appearance, it is not surprising that such women would go to any length to be thin and attractive. They diet (and binge and purge) and exercise and dress with the constant compulsion to be as thin and beautiful as possible. Our current standard of beauty, which includes extreme slenderness, provides an added burden for many bulimic women, especially those whose bodies were never meant to be so thin.

It saddens and angers me to see young girls of fourteen or fifteen (at an age when their bodies really need food) dieting themselves to semistarvation to meet our culture's unrealistically thin body standards, just so they can be attractive to boys. During these years, the years in which their self-concepts and their sense of self-worth are forming, they are learning from television, popular magazines, and romantic novels, that their job in life is to be attractive (read thin). These girls are bulimics and anorectics in the making.

Most adult bulimic women also have distorted body images. Often a woman will come into my office, complaining of weight gain. "This is the heaviest I've ever been in my life," she may say. All I see is a woman who is fashionably, in some cases even painfully, thin. Though the world may not view them as fat, they view themselves so, and look with horror at each new pound of fat. Fat phobia, though it is largely ignored by doctors and therapists who view these women as normal weights who do not really have a problem, needs to be taken seriously. The extra pound may mean more to a woman with bulimia than twenty or thirty pounds will to an obese woman. It is unfortunate that the complaints of bulimic women are not taken seriously. These women truly feel fat. The work for such patients includes determining the origins and function of their fat phobia, as well as working on and correcting their distorted body image. For those of you who are bulimic, the chapter on "Bodywork" will be most useful in helping you to readjust your body image to a more realistic standard. Chapter 2, "The Power of Fat" will help you discover more about the symbolic meanings fat may have for you and what you can do about it.

At this point, it will be necessary to caution those of you who are bulimic that though my book will be helpful in giving you some insight into your eating problem, the book alone is not enough. Bulimia is a more serious eating disorder than simple compulsive eating or overweight and requires treatment with a competent, trained psychotherapist. I cannot stress enough the need for therapy in overcoming this disorder. Your first consideration in choosing a therapist would be in finding someone, male or female, who is nonsexist and will not reinforce your belief that you *need* to be attractive. It is also important that the therapist be aware of or, even better, specifically trained in the treatment of bulimic women. Traditional psychotherapy, while helpful in many respects, has not been successful in treating bulimia (or most eating disorders, for that matter). Physicians and psychotherapists have tended to make light of the problem, since most bulimic women are of normal weight, as though the degree of severity of an eating disorder can be measured by body weight.

Some traditional therapists, while aware of the severity of the eating disorder, have looked at the disordered eating behavior as symptomatic of an underlying emotional problem and have chosen to ignore the symptom, treating the underlying problems and expecting the symptom (the disordered eating behaviors) to disappear as the underlying problems were worked through. Such treatment has been ineffective, and though such patients have shown improvement in their self-esteem and exhibit lowered levels of anxiety and depression, their bulimic eating patterns remain. Therefore, it is necessary to find a therapist who will work with you on the eating behaviors as well—who has training in dealing with this specific problem. If you are unable to locate such a therapist, try contacting your local hospital or mental health service. Many hospitals have begun setting up eating disorder clinics. You can also write to ANAD (Anorexia Nervosa and Associated Disorders), a nonprofit group which will send you a list of therapists in your area who are able to treat bulimia. Send a stamped, self-addressed business-sized envelope ($.35 postage) to ANAD, Suite 2020, 550 Frontage Rd., Northfield, IL 60093. They also have a hotline: (312) 831-3438.

Though I am stressing the need for psychotherapy, I still feel this book can be useful to you in gaining some understanding of the dynamics and underlying causes of your problem, and if used in conjunction with therapy can provide a framework within which to view your eating disorder. As I continue to discuss the issues associated with bulimia, I will point out which chapters of the book can be utilized to help you deal with your problems.

Let us now turn our attention to the binges which accompany this disorder. It is an assumption of my approach to eating problems that the binges, as self-destructive as they may seem on the surface, are serving a function for the bulimic woman (as well as for most compulsive eaters). Rather than trying to control those binges, an effort which leads almost inevitably to failure, the work presented here will focus on determining the purpose of these binges. Perhaps some examples will best explain this concept.

Let us take the case of Beth. She has been in treatment for a short time and still views her binges as a sign of lack of control: "If I could only exert enough control over my eating, I'd be okay. I can string three, four good days together, and then I explode, eating everything in sight." She wants me to help her bolster her self-control so that the binges will no longer occur. What she doesn't yet realize is that those binges are not accidents, and not evidence of any lack of self-imposed discipline, but result from inner, unconscious needs to use food and eating. Beth is not consciously aware of her motivations to binge, and the first step in her treatment is to become aware of why she might actually be *wanting* to binge (on some level) — what needs she is using the binges to meet. Through the use of a guided fantasy in which the food "talks" to Beth (this fantasy is explained in detail in Chapter 6, "The Power of Food"), she is able to discover that the binges do indeed have a function in her life. She learns that by stuffing herself with food, she is blocking out all awareness of her feelings. All she feels is the physical pain caused by overeating and vomiting. Binging allows her to refocus her attention from painful emotions and thoughts to eating and physical discomfort. It is actually easier for Beth to deal with the binging, and the emotional and physical discomfort it causes, than to deal with what is really bothering her.

In this context, the aftermath of a binge—the anger at oneself, the frustration, depression, and self-disgust—can be viewed as serving a dual function. First of all, it may be more acceptable and easier for the bulimic to direct her self-disgust and anger toward her inability to control her eating than toward herself in general. Having such high standards for herself, the bulimic woman often feels she has fallen short of what she "should" be. Rather than feel the self-disgust and frustration at her inability to live up to her standards, she may displace the feelings into her problem with food. Then the negative feelings and self-judgments can be assuaged by embarking on a new diet, which brings us to the second function of the binge. She gives herself a way out of those feelings—a path to salvation. All she need do is reassert control and go on a diet, and she will feel better about herself.

The next step in treatment is to become aware of the specific feelings the bulimic woman is trying to avoid by focusing on the binge. In Beth's case it might be anger that constantly triggers a binge. In exploring Beth's background, we discover that she has always been a "good girl," has always seen her role in life as pleasing others. This view of herself, fostered by her parents, made it very difficult for Beth to learn to deal with anger. Anger, to Beth, represents a threat. "People won't be happy with me if I get angry at them or I provoke anger in them. They won't love me or even like me." Her fear of anger became so strong that she learned to block all awareness of angry feelings. In her mind, they do not exist. "I *never* get angry," she would proclaim. The only anger she allowed herself to feel was at herself, and that was directed primarily at her binges. What Beth was doing during her binges was stuffing down anger by refocusing her attention from inner feelings to food and eating. In addition, she displaced her anger at others onto herself, hating herself for what she viewed as her self-destructive eating behavior. Beth's work in treatment would consist in exploring anger—what it means to her, what she fears—and in learning to express it verbally. She would also need to focus on the way she has used food to "stuff down" the angry feelings. In essence, she has been giving food the power to suppress angry feelings, but food cannot do that. Food is not a drug. The concept of how food is being used to meet emotional needs and what you can do about it is the subject of the chapter "The Power of Food."

Anger was also connected to the binges of another woman with whom I worked—Helen. In this case, Helen's husband was aware of her bulimic behavior. She had told him. The binging and subsequent purges disturbed her husband so much that Helen was able to use them as a weapon against him. Helen was also unable to express anger directly (though unlike Beth, she was aware of her angry feelings at her husband) and so she expressed her anger indirectly, through her eating. Whenever she felt angry with her husband, Helen would binge and vomit for hours, making sure he was aware of what was happening. If he were not home at the time, she would leave evidence around, indicating that a binge had taken place—empty pie plates, crumbs, plates on her nighttable.

I must emphasize that Helen was only partially aware of the motivations underlying her behavior. Occasionally during a binge, she would have thoughts of "I'll show him," but for the most part, she had no conscious awareness of why she needed to binge. Her awareness that her binges were serving to express anger at her husband came from examining the circumstances surrounding the binges. I had asked her to keep a journal of her binges, recording the events, thoughts, and feelings that preceded them and the thoughts, if any, that she was aware of during the binge. After several weeks, a pattern began to emerge. She began to see that her binges almost always were precipitated by an incident with her husband which provoked an angry response within her. She would soon find herself, as though in a trance, going into the kitchen or out to buy food in order to binge; and she would always leave evidence, seemingly inadvertent, of her binge and purge, as though she wanted him to know about it. She realized that her binges and the vomiting disturbed her husband greatly, and that on some level, she was using the eating behavior to get back at him. Her work with me consisted in learning to express her anger more directly, and as she began to do so, the frequency of her binges decreased dramatically.

Another patient of mine, Barbara, discovered her binges were serving a function in her life, as well. Barbara was a seventeen-year-old college freshman. She came from a well-to-do family in which both parents were professionals—her mother an accountant, her father a lawyer. The youngest of three children (the other two of whom were studying law), Barbara felt an enormous pressure to achieve. She was extremely intelligent and capable, but her temperament was not suited to a high-pressure career, and she would have been happy to become a wife and mother. Instead, she was pushing herself to study law, like her sister and brother, ignoring her rather strong needs to relax, to pull back and enjoy life. What Barbara discovered was that her eating disorder—the binges and the purges and the concentration of enormous amounts of energy and time on the problem—allowed her to escape her high expectations of herself: "How much can I expect to do when I spend all day binging?" she would say, seemingly annoyed at herself, but secretly relieved that the pressure to achieve was off. Very often she would binge merely to allow herself the luxury of staying home.

Another patient, Susan, came to see that her binges served to isolate her from others, but in a protective way. She felt pressure to "be out there in the world." It was not okay with her to spend a day at home, away from friends and family. She lived in a very wealthy, socially-oriented environment. Despite her beliefs about the importance of getting out of the house and socializing, Susan had a strong need to be alone sometimes—to get away from people. She came to realize that her binges allowed her to stay at home and be by herself. She discovered this function of the binges by asking herself one day while eating: "What am I using this binge for? What is it I *really* want?" The answer came from deep inside her: "I am binging today so that I don't have to go to a meeting with my friends. I really just want to stay home alone. If I'm on a binge, I won't have to go." Susan had to face up to her need to be alone occasionally in order to give up her binges. She had to allow for that part of her which needed to be alone. Susan also binged when she needed to isolate herself from her immediate family. She became so wrapped up in her eating and purging, she felt as though she were alone or at least apart from the people around her.

Binges can also function as a defense against anxiety and depression, and, as we learned earlier in this chapter, bulimic women tend to exhibit higher than normal levels of both anxiety and depression. They may use food to allay anxiety, as though it were a tranquilizer. The intense concentration of energy on planning binges, on eating, and on purging can serve to focus attention away from anxious or depressed feelings. One of my patients stated: "As painful as my eating problem is, it is still easier for me to deal with the binging and vomiting than with depression." The fear, on some level, is "If I don't eat, I'll be overwhelmed with anxiety or fall into a deep depression."

As difficult as it may be to accept, the binges and vomiting of bulimia may function as a way of being good to oneself. The bulimic woman is being good to herself in the sense that she is taking into herself something she loves—food. The vomiting can be viewed as a way of giving to herself in that she is making sure she will not suffer the consequences of enjoying that food, that she will not gain weight. In such a case, it would be necessary to look at that woman's life and try to discover what is lacking that she needs to "give" to herself in such a way. Is she giving to herself materially, emotionally, spiritually, in other ways? If not, why not? Is she giving out so much of herself to others that the only pleasure she takes in is food?

The binges of another of my patients, Ana, were related to the issue of control. Ana often binged when she felt out of control over what was happening to her. When her life was going well, and she felt able to handle all the problems which arose, Ana had no trouble keeping her eating "under control," but if a day went poorly, if things began to happen over which she felt she had no control (her child getting sick, the doctor canceling an appointment, a car breaking down) Ana would turn to food, eating everything she could find. Her eating would go "out of control" along with the rest of her life. Ana had two views of herself: "in control of everything" or "out of control over everything." There was no concept of an Ana, confronted with little and big life crises, out of control over the circumstances and perhaps outcomes of those crises, but still eating "normally." Ana's experience is a common one.

The issue of control is crucial to the understanding of bulimia; It is one of the major factors in the life of a bulimic woman. As I see it, there are many factors involved, and perhaps if we explore each factor separately, you can gain a deeper understanding of the issue of control and how it is associated with the binging and purging behavior. A case history might provide a vehicle by which this matter of control can be best understood. Using Ana's case as an example, let us turn to the origins of the need to feel in control.

Ana, like many bulimic women, was brought up to be a "good girl." She was "daddy's girl," though she was close to her mother as well. Encouraged by her father, she learned to be sweet and pleasing as a way of getting what she wanted from others. She began to feel that the only way to get what she wanted in the world and the only way to get love was by pleasing people all the time. Negative emotions—anger, frustration, disappointment in others—were unacceptable to her, because by feeling them she risked antagonizing or disturbing another. Only positive, loving emotions were allowed. To Ana, angering someone else meant losing their love. So Ana learned to repress those emotions, keeping them out of awareness. Such repression required an enormous effort of control, as Ana had to monitor and censor everything she felt before she allowed it into her consciousness. It took every ounce of her strength to maintain this vigilant control over herself, and though to the outside world she seemed a sweet, loving, even-tempered person, she appeared so only at great cost to herself. Ana, unaware of what she was trying to control within herself, knew only that she must be vigilant in monitoring herself, and she often panicked at the thought of losing control. She had no idea what she was afraid she would lose control of, but she thought that if she let go, something terrible would happen to her. This need for control was projected outside her as well, as she had a desperate need to be in control of everything in her life. Out of touch with so many of her emotions, Ana became increasingly out of touch with her body. And though she was hypersensitive to whatever physical sensations were taking place within her, she did not trust her body because her body was not under the control of her rational conscious mind. More and more aspects of her life came under control as she got older. By the time she had reached adulthood, Ana could not even trust herself to regulate her food intake. Decisions about what to eat, when, and how much were conscious intellectual judgments about what was "right" rather than responses to signals her body was sending about its food needs.

"How was this issue of control reflected in Ana's eating problem?" you might ask. The manifestations were many. Ana's strict diets were a form of rigid control over what she viewed as her "instinctual, unpredictable body." Concentrating on obtaining the "correct" foods in the "proper" amounts gave a structure to her day, as well, and a sense that she was "in control." The binges allowed her to escape from that rigid control. Though it was much too frightening a prospect to let go of the control she exerted over her emotional self, Ana had created a situation in which she let go on a limited basis. She set up a strict diet which she maintained for some time, and then she would rebel. She would break loose, eating everything she could find. She *felt* out of control but in fact was *going* "out of control" in a controlled way. It was only in this area of her life that this rebellious, uncontrollable behavior occurred. Clearly, she could face the pain of letting go with respect to eating more easily than letting go in her whole emotional self. The binges provided a limited outlet for the tension she created in her constant vigilance over herself. The subsequent self-induced vomiting gave her the sense of reestablishing control—determining what would remain or not remain in her body.

The binges also served to hold down negative emotions, especially anger, since Ana felt the food was stuffing them down. Usually unaware that she was angry at someone, she was conscious only of anxious feelings and would quickly reach for food to make them go away. She would stuff food in her mouth as though food really had the power to hold down emotions. Actually, the binges served to refocus her attention away from the feelings threatening to break through, onto the binge. The self-hate, self-disgust, and frustration were less painful, less threatening emotions than negative feelings toward another person.

Treatment for women such as Ana focuses on this issue of control, as well as many other important issues associated with the bulimia. A typical treatment program would include the following:

1. Exploring the origins of the patient's problem with control. This aspect of the work includes a detailed family history and an examination of how the patient came to feel the need to exert so great a control over herself.
2. The use of imagery and body awareness exercises to help the woman get back in touch with her bodily sensations. As we have seen, most bulimic women do not trust their bodies because they view so many of the body's functions as outside their conscious control (Chapter 4, "Bodywork," deals with body awareness).
3. Learning to respond to the body's normal sensations of hunger in determining eating behavior, rather than to a self-imposed intellectual control over the eating process. Once the bulimic woman has gained some trust in her physical sensations, attention can be turned to learning about the sensations which signal the body's food needs. The woman can learn to follow her body's messages in determining what, when, and how much food is needed. The sense of control is therefore internalized, rather than dependent on external authorities or controls. Your body knows best what it needs. This aspect of the work is extremely difficult for most bulimics. They fear giving up conscious control over their eating and trusting their bodies to tell them what they need. However, it is only by giving up dieting and learning to eat out of physical need that the dieting-binging-purging cycle can be broken permanently. ("Eating Awareness," Chapter 5, deals with this topic in detail.)
4. Exploring the functions that binging and purging serve in the woman's life, and helping her find new ways of fulfilling those functions other than through the use of food. As we have seen, the binges may serve many functions in a bulimic woman's life, though on the surface they may seem merely self-destructive acts. Once these functions have been uncovered, new ways can

be found to meet those needs. It is important to gain an understanding of what one has been using the food to do, so that other ways of satisfying those needs can be found. (Chapter 6, "The Power of Food," will help you gain insight into how food and the binges and purges are functioning in your life.)

5. Correcting distorted body images. Women who are bulimic often view themselves as much heavier than they really are. Work is done on exploring the origins and functions of this distorted body image. (Chapter 4 on "Bodywork" focuses on body image.)

6. Finding the weight at which the woman is most comfortable: in some cases, a woman's body weight may be somewhat higher than her present weight (which may be unrealistically low and which may be causing emotional and physical stress on the body). As difficult as it may seem, it is *sometimes* necessary for a bulimic woman actually to gain a few pounds. (Chapter 7, "Putting It All Together," deals with the topic of finding the most comfortable weight and provides you with some of the most recent research findings on weight and dieting.)

7. Relaxation training. Because the anxiety level of most bulimic women is so high, and because binges often function to allay anxiety, some training in relaxation techniques is often necessary. Some of the women with whom I work take up yoga or biofeedback or meditation.

8. Assertiveness training. Unable to feel or express anger and other negative emotions, and feeling controlled by the expectations and desires of others, many women with bulimia lack the skills necessary to assert their needs and desires. Learning to assert themselves effectively is part of the process of giving up their eating problem, since so often binges occur when the bulimic woman fails to express her feelings directly and openly to another.

9. Exploring and developing the woman's sense of self-esteem. The bulimic woman needs to explore her dependence on others, especially men, in determining how she feels about herself. She needs to feel in control of her self-image and sense of self-worth. She has to learn to act out of her own needs, rather than those of another.

10. Finally, learning to accept herself—her good and bad characteristics, her strengths and her weaknesses. (The sense of nonjudgmental awareness and acceptance of oneself pervades every chapter of the book.)

Remember that this book alone will not be enough to bring you along on your journey in recovering from bulimia. It is my strong belief that professional help is also necessary, but the insights gained from reading this book may help you greatly in gaining a new perspective on your problem. The steps I have just outlined, as well as the chapters dealing with each specific topic, can provide you with a framework within which to view your treatment.

The road to a life without bulimia is not an easy one. Much work needs to be done, but with a commitment, a decision to face whatever has to be faced, you can do it. I know. I did.

two

The Power of Fat

Fat is serving many functions in your life. You may on all conscious levels hate it, but on a deeper, subconscious level, you have given fat the power to do something, many things, for you. You have learned to adapt to circumstances in your life and meet certain needs by getting fat and eating compulsively. In this chapter, you will discover how fat is functioning in your life, what powers you have given to fat and how you can take this power back.

What is meant by the "power of fat"? An illustration will provide the clearest explanation. Let us take the common complaint: "Fat keeps me home, it keeps me from going out." Fat does not keep one from going out. Fat does not *do* anything. It is one's attitudes about the fat which determine the behavior. In order to give up her fat, the woman voicing this complaint must realize that it is *she* who keeps herself home, all the while attributing the decision to fat. In other words, she *gives fat the power* to keep her home. Next, this woman must begin exploring the possibility that she does not really *want* to go out, or at least is ambivalent about leaving. Maybe a part of her enjoys being home alone, but another part says she "ought" to go out or should be more active and involved with other people. A more accurate statement might read, "I use my fat as an excuse to stay home."

It is not enough, though, to identify what powers one has given to fat. In order to lose weight permanently, one must take that power back. I have come to believe that there is a dynamic process, a course one follows in learning to take this power back. The process can be broken down into steps, though not everyone will follow every step for every problem, nor will the order of these steps remain static. Yet it is helpful to keep this concept of a process in mind and use the description presented here as a guideline on your own journey. The general outline will prove helpful in allowing you to make use of the information obtained in the various exercises in this chapter. The process consists of:

1. Uncovering and identifying the functions fat has been serving for you both in the past and present. In other words, *"What* have I given the fat the power to do for me?" The directed fantasies and other mental exercises in this chapter aim at uncovering this largely subconscious material.
2. Determining *why* you have chosen to use fat to meet your needs. "Why did I give the power to fat in the first place?" This step may also involve an examination of past as well as present experiences.
3. Exploring why you might not *want* to take the power back from the fat.
4. Realizing that it is not the fat (in most cases) which is "doing anything" for you.
5. Seeking and trying out new ways to meet your needs other than through fat. In other words, *"How* can I take the power back from the fat?" This last step, the most difficult one, is a most important part of the process. It requires you to actually *do* something with the self-knowledge you have obtained.

To best understand this process, I will present the case of a hypothetical patient. We will trace her progress from the discovery of one of the functions her fat has been serving to her search for new ways to meet her needs without the fat.

Let us call her Jennifer. Jennifer is a married woman in her middle thirties, with dark black hair and deep, dark brown eyes. On her 5'2" frame, she carries 160 pounds, and she is miserable with herself. Having tried for years to reduce, she has come to me, not necessarily because she believes her problem to be psychological, but because I am presenting yet another method to get thin. She is somewhat skeptical when she hears me say that the fat is helping her in some ways—that she is using it to perform some functions for her. In fact, she maintains, "There's no possible use for this blob. I'm fat because I love to eat and I have no will power."

She initially endures my proclamations about the functions of fat with skepticism, and remains in treatment only because her neighbor had lost fifty pounds while in one of my groups.

Then one day, during her third group session, Jennifer tries one of the guided visualizations aimed at uncovering her unconscious associations with fat, and she discovers much to her surprise that she has been using her fat to "keep men away." The realization of what she has given the fat the power to do is but a first step. The questions now arise: Why did she have to give the power to the fat in the first place? Why does she want to keep men away, and why does she have to use *fat* to do so?

We may find that Jennifer has always been a somewhat submissive, nonassertive woman, who has difficulty saying "no," especially to men. As a young woman she may have found herself involved in sexual situations or relationships for which she was ill-prepared or which she did not desire, solely because of her inability to say "no." Such women are not uncommon in our society. Women are neither trained nor encouraged (rather they are discouraged) to assert themselves directly. A large part of Jennifer's difficulty in saying "no" to men results because: 1) she has not learned to say "no" gracefully and in a way she feels comfortable with; and 2) she is always thinking about the other person's needs and does not want to hurt the man's feelings. So, she finds herself going out with, sleeping with and possibly (as in some extreme cases) marrying a man she does not love, because rejecting him would hurt his feelings. At this point, Jennifer might begin to see how she chose, at least on an unconscious level, to give her power to fat: Fat would keep men away. Fat would say "no" for her. Fat would allow her to avoid uncomfortable situations. To take responsibility for herself would have meant saying "no," but because she could not say "no" to men, she had to attribute the power to some "outside" force—the fat. As to why she has been reluctant to take this power back from the fat, to do so would be to place herself in a position she has neither learned to deal with nor feels capable of handling.

In addition, there might be another function tied up with the fat, which Jennifer would discover upon further exploration of her problem. There may also be a part of her which does not *want* to say "no" to sexual encounters. She may fantasize about having affairs, even though the thought of acting on these fantasies actually scares her. She may consider that part of her which desires extramarital sexual contact to be her promiscuous side, a part of her which could take control over her behavior. She may also consider the fat as her primary means of keeping her promiscuous longings under control. "How could I have an affair when I'm so fat? No man would be interested in me, and even if he were, I'd be too ashamed for him to see my body." She might even have a particular man in mind and would fear "as soon as I lost the weight, I'd call him up on the phone." To lose the fat would mean losing the only thing she perceives as holding her back — restraining her from acting on impulses about which she feels ambivalent, at best.

The next step for Jennifer would likely be a more difficult one to take, for it requires her to begin taking the power back from the fat — it is the realization that it is not the *fat* which has kept men away or even that it has kept her promiscuous side under control. At this point, Jennifer might protest. "I can see how I've been using my fat to protect me, but it *is* the fat which keeps me from getting involved with men. Men in our culture are turned off by fat women." To an extent, this notion is true but even if a woman has so much fat on her body that most men would be "turned off," she is still relying on some outside force — as she perceives it — to keep men away. In such a case, the woman still does not own the power to define her own sexuality and to set limits on her sexual encounters. She gives her power to her fat.

To repeat, *it is not the fat itself which keeps men away*. In part, it is the woman's attitude toward her fat and her body to which most men respond. I have seen several women who, though overweight by any standards, were considered sexy, womanly, and extremely attractive. I have also seen women with whom I have worked develop a sense of sexual worth and beauty, develop a "presence" to which men and women alike are often attracted.

I do not expect to have convinced you entirely yet as to my position, as surely I would not have convinced Jennifer. So, I would ask her at this point to observe the interactions of other women and men—both in her own life, and in the movies, television, and novels she reads. I would ask her to observe how a woman lets a man know she is not interested.

Jennifer might then begin to realize that there are many ways, verbal and nonverbal, in which women can express their sexual interest in men and at the same time set limits on their interactions with them. She might become aware of the nonverbal messages—clothes, the way you hold your body, eye contact, touch or lack of it—which convey to a man "I'm sexy. I think you are too," or "Stay away. I'm not interested."

At the same time, I would want to work with Jennifer on her belief that it is the fat alone which is keeping her from having an affair. I might tell her that, no matter how happily married a woman might be, it is perfectly normal to have fantasies and longings for extramarital sexual contact. Whether one chooses to act on them or not is another matter; but the important point is that there is a choice, a choice Jennifer has already made, though she does not realize it. If she has not had an affair yet, it is not because of her fat, but *because she has ambivalent feelings about acting out her fantasies*. She has kept herself from becoming involved with another man because of her fears or her moral judgments of such behavior. Yet she maintains, "It is fat which holds me back," ignoring her fears and negative feelings about such "promiscuous behavior." She might have to accept on faith, at least at first, that you will not do anything for which you are not ready. You do not have to give up your fat until you are ready. On the other hand, you can get thin and still leave unresolved your desires for an affair. You can be thin and still be ambivalent about taking action. You can be thin and *not* have an affair, if you want.

Jennifer must begin to disengage her fat from all other problems in her life—to realize that she can have a problem with her sexuality, for example, fat or thin. She must begin to see her difficulties with her sexuality as problems in their own right, not necessarily tied inextricably to her fat. Jennifer's difficulties with men, with her sexuality, and with assertion would not disappear were she to lose weight. On the other hand, she need not get thin to overcome these difficulties.

Once Jennifer begins making the separation between her fat and other problems in her life, she enters the final stage of the process—taking the power back from the fat. Jennifer now knows what powers she has attributed to the fat, how the fat has functioned in her life, and why she chose to give the power to fat in the first place. Yet, she may complain, "I'm still eating. I'm still fat. Where has all this self-knowledge gotten me?" And I would patiently explain that, while the self-knowledge is important, indeed necessary, it is not enough. There is another step to be taken, one which is equally as important and usually more difficult to accomplish—*doing* something with the knowledge you have acquired.

In Jennifer's case, "doing something" might entail, first of all, learning to say "no" to a man in a manner with which she will feel comfortable. Her difficulty with assertion may extend to other areas of her life, and I would recommend a good assertiveness training course, or we would work in group on establishing new assertive behaviors.

At the same time, Jennifer might be working on redefining her sexuality. Instead of viewing her sexuality as tied up to her body weight and defined by the men she meets, she would finally learn control over the sexual messages she puts out and those she chooses to withhold. Such learning comes through experimentation, reflection, and then more experimentation. The experience of one of my patients, Rita, may illustrate what I mean by experimentation, since she was involved, while in her group, in trying out such new behaviors. During one group session she described an incident in which she allowed herself to enjoy a sexual interaction with a man, at the same time setting limits on their encounter. By "sexual interaction" it should be pointed out that I do not necessarily mean sexual intercourse. There are a whole range of interactions between human beings which can be labeled sexual, and, as many women are beginning to learn, sharing a "sexual" experience with another person does not necessarily lead to going to bed with that person.

Rita had been riding in a crowded commuter railroad train. The seats in her car were placed in such a manner that it would be difficult to avoid knocking knees with the person sitting opposite. She noticed a man sitting across from her whom she found particularly attractive, and who seemed to find her so as well. She gave him direct eye contact for a few seconds and then broke it off abruptly. They spent the rest of the trip knocking knees (more than would be expected) and fantasizing in their heads about what they would have liked to be doing together. When she reached her stop, Rita got up from her seat, they smiled at each other ever so slightly, and Rita left the train. Not a word had been spoken.

In this one small incident Rita learned many things: that she was a sexually attractive woman even at what she considered a heavy weight, that she could interact "sexually" in a way she saw fit, and that *she* could set the limits on her interactions with a man. Rita set her limits by choosing what appeared to be a safe man—a suburban commuter on his way home from work—in a safe place—a crowded train. She also set a limit by making eye contact briefly and then cutting it off abruptly, implying, "I'm interested, but not in *too* much." Her experience convinced her, more than any of our discussions on the subject, that she was in control of her sexual interactions with men. Jennifer is in need of just such experience. Jennifer needs to actually experience this sense of control and to realize that the control comes from within and does not reside wholly outside her or in her fat. Once she owns this power for herself, the fat can be lost.

I wish I could report that having completed this process of taking the power back from the fat, Jennifer would go on to lose all her weight and live happily ever after (as most diet books would have you believe), but such would not necessarily be the case. We have explored in this example only one major function the fat has been serving in her life. There may be many other functions to work through as well, but with respect to each, the process would remain the same.

At first, it may seem discouraging to discover that you may have given power to your fat to meet so many needs. The task of identifying all the functions the fat has been serving, and the process of taking the power back from the fat, may appear overwhelming. But do not be discouraged. The work ahead is not as difficult as it appears. Perhaps the following explanation will help.

I sometimes envision the fat problem as a tangled web: a ball wrapped in string represents the fat at the center, and radiating out in all directions are strings, masses of strings, attached to many problem areas in a woman's life. For example, let us take the case of Sara. While in her group, she mapped out the following diagram to illustrate how her fat was related to other problems:

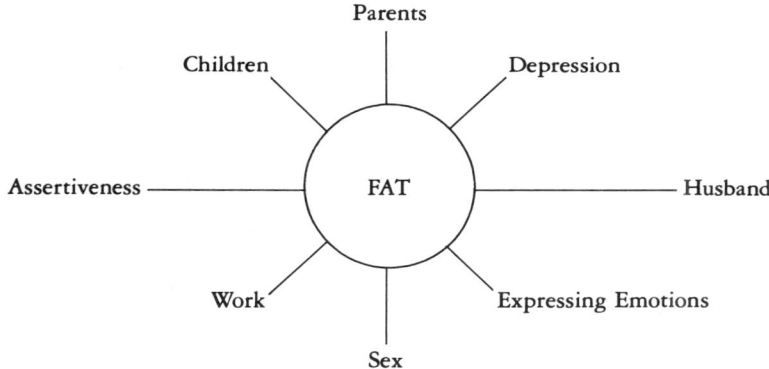

As you can see from the diagram, Sara's fat is connected to nearly everything she experiences, and treatment would consist, in part, of cutting those strings, one by one—disconnecting the fat from each problem area, so that the fat can be lost permanently. The problem areas may remain unresolved. Sara may still have difficulties with sex and her emotions. Her relationship with her parents and children may still be fraught with troubles. Yet her fat will no longer be the issue; it will no longer be tied to how well or how poorly she is doing in dealing with those problems. The process of cutting those ties between fat and all one's other problems is a long but manageable one. You can get thin without resolving completely all the problem areas to which your fat is connected. All that is necessary is that you *break* those connections.

The remainder of this chapter provides you with the tools to break these connections, to uncover the functions fat has been serving, and to guide you in the process of taking the power back from the fat.

Let us begin with a brief introduction to the guided fantasies or directed visualizations, as they are sometimes called. The guided fantasies presented here are tools which may enable you to tap the resources of your subconscious mind. They are the means whereby you can gain awareness of thoughts, feelings, emotions, and memories that you are not conscious of during your normal waking state of mind. A typical guided fantasy might require you to relax deeply, then to imagine yourself in a situation in which you are as thin as you would ever like to be. I might ask that you be aware of how you feel in this thin body, what you are wearing, if anything about being this thin makes you feel uncomfortable, and so on. Very often the reactions are surprising. These fantasies do not feel very different from the daydreams we all experience from time to time, except that instead of arising spontaneously in your mind, the situations and circumstances of the fantasy are created *for* you. (Hence the term "directed" or "guided" fantasies.)

Many people fear such experiences as a form of control by another, but they are nothing of the sort. When you take a fantasy trip, you are not under the control of anyone other than yourself. Though someone may suggest the circumstances, set the stage, so to speak, it is you and you alone who write the script. There are others who fear contact with their subconscious, fear that they will lose control. This is not so, particularly in the case of the fantasies presented in this book. It is important to realize that you will not find out anything you do not want to know or with which you are not ready to deal. You will protect yourself either by having trouble concentrating, and thereby not being able to "get into" the fantasy, or by forgetting or not understanding what occurred. However, if you ever find yourself particularly disturbed by something you have discovered as a result of creating one of these fantasies, by all means talk about it with someone you trust. It is unlikely that such an experience will prove to be any more upsetting than a disturbing dream.

Usually a fantasy is preceded by a short relaxation period. You may use any of the relaxation exercises from this book, or you may spend a few minutes relaxing in any other manner you have learned. Biofeedback techniques, yoga, and self hypnosis are all helpful. The greater your state of relaxation, the more clearly and distinctly you will be able to visualize and "get into" the fantasy. The more you "get into" it, the more you will get out of it.

I suggest that, if possible, you tape the fantasies beforehand, or have someone read them to you, as it is quite disrupting to have to open your eyes repeatedly to read what comes next. The dots between sentences represent pauses of five to ten seconds. Be sure to leave plenty of time during those pauses to allow yourself to develop your images to the fullest. Longer pauses are indicated in the text of each fantasy.

Each guided fantasy will be followed by a discussion of the experiences and insights of some of the women who have tried the fantasy, as well as a guideline to help you analyze your own experience. I suggest, however, that you not attempt to analyze or interpret your fantasies while you are doing them—just let each one develop, without planning or censorship. Analysis and interpretation are best left for the period afterward.

RELAXATION EXERCISES

Choose one of the following exercises or any other with which you are familiar, and spend five to ten minutes relaxing before each fantasy.

#1

Sit or lie comfortably . . . close your eyes and relax . . . Imagine that relaxing energy is entering your body through your head. . . . As this energy passes through each part of your body, you feel the muscles loosen, and all tension leaves the area. . . . Begin to feel your scalp relax . . . and your forehead. . . . Feel your eyes yield to this calming energy . . . and your cheeks . . . your mouth . . . your jaw. . . . Let the tension leave your neck . . . shoulders . . . arms. . . . Feel your chest relaxing . . . your stomach . . . back. . . . Feel the muscles in your buttocks go slack . . . relax your pelvic area . . . your hips . . . thighs . . . legs, all the way down to your toes. (Pause fifteen seconds.) . . . Let the relaxing energy flow through your body, allowing you to feel completely relaxed and comfortable. (Pause thirty seconds). . . . Let your body go limp, as you let the muscles relax completely. . . . (Pause two minutes.)

#2

Lie down and close your eyes. . . . Imagine yourself floating on a puffy white cloud. . . . Just relax and enjoy the pleasant feeling of floating. (Pause fifteen seconds.) . . . As you float on the cloud a pleasant feeling of comfort and peace comes over you. . . . You can feel your body becoming very relaxed as you float . . . gently . . . freely. . . . You notice the deep blue sky, as you float comfortably on this cloud. . . . The sun shines warmly on your face . . . and you can feel a gentle breeze blowing. (Pause twenty seconds.) . . . All the noise and bustle of the everyday world is far away, and all around you is peace and calmness. (Pause fifteen seconds.) . . . There is nothing to worry about and nothing to do, so just relax and enjoy the pleasantness of floating on this cloud. . . . (Pause two minutes.)

#3

Find a comfortable position and close your eyes. . . . Become aware of any tensions in your body, and just relax them. (Pause twenty seconds.) . . . Imagine that each of your tensions and worries is a balloon . . . a balloon filled with helium. . . . One by one, each balloon rises up to the sky, taking with it a problem, a source of worry and tension. (Pause fifteen seconds.) . . . As you watch each balloon rise, you feel less and less burdened with troubles and more and more relaxed and free. . . . If it makes you feel more comfortable knowing you are not giving up your problems forever, imagine all the balloons collecting in one place, each attached to a string firmly tied to the ground. . . . Whenever you want these troubles back again you need only pull the string. . . . In the meantime, feel wonderfully relaxed and free, knowing that, at least temporarily, your tensions and worries are gone. (Pause two minutes.) . . .

PREFACE TO GUIDE FANTASY[1]

The first fantasy I wish to present is not limited in its applicability to discovering the functions fat has been serving in your life. As a matter of fact, the guide fantasy is the most powerful and useful one I have ever used, both personally and professionally. Once a relationship has been established with your guide, access to your own natural wisdom is assured, and a limitless store of information and knowledge is as close as a "trip" inside your mind. Let us make it clear from the start that the guide you are about to meet is none other than yourself—a part of yourself which arises in your subconscious and which allows you access to the treasury of wisdom to be found within. This fantasy gives form to this part of yourself—personifies it—and though I am asking you to talk to another "person," remember she is really you.

Before you begin, think of a question concerning your eating or weight to which you especially want an answer. You might ask why you are holding onto your fat or what fears you have about being thin. You may want to know what you have to do to enable yourself to lose your fat premanently. Whatever the question, the answers are inside you.[2]

THE GUIDE

Close your eyes and imagine yourself in a beautiful peaceful place—somewhere you have been before, or somewhere you would like to be. . . . Try to make the image of this place as vivid as possible. . . . Be aware of your surroundings . . . the sounds . . . the colors . . . the smells . . . the sights around you. . . . Just relax and enjoy the peacefulness and pleasantness of this beautiful place. Spend a few minutes enjoying yourself. (Pause at least one minute.)

Now, still envisioning yourself in this beautiful, comfortable place, I want you to become aware of your breathing. . . . Imagine that as you inhale, a stream of relaxing energy is entering your body, and as you exhale, the energy leaves your body, taking with it all tensions, worries, and troubles (pause fifteen seconds) . . .

with each exhalation you feel more and more relaxed. (Pause fifteen seconds). . . . Continue breathing this way, envisioning yourself in this beautiful and peaceful place for a few minutes. (Pause at least two minutes.)

Now, still envisioning yourself in this beautiful, comfortable place, look around you and you will become aware of the presence of a living being. . . . You may not actually see her yet, but somehow you will sense her presence (pause fifteen seconds). . . . Somehow you will sense the presence of a loving, accepting wise woman. (Pause thirty seconds.) You may begin to see her more clearly now, or you may just continue to sense that she is with you, but either way you will sense her loving and caring and wisdom (pause fifteen seconds). . . . This woman is your guide, your advisor, a link with your subconscious. She is the part of you who knows the answers to all your questions. Spend some time getting to know her. . . . Ask her name. . . . Tell her yours. . . . Walk with her a bit. . . . She is to become your friend and advisor, so spend some time finding out who she is and how she lives. . . . (Pause one minute.)

Ask your guide what she wants from you in return for her help . . . (pause fifteen seconds). . . . Now, I would like you to ask your guide some question which is especially important to you, a question which concerns your weight or your eating (pause twenty seconds). . . . Your guide may answer with words alone, or she may show you a picture or a gesture. She may give you something —but in *some* way she is going to give you the answer to your question (pause one minute). . . . If you do not understand your guide's answer, ask her to explain . . . ask her to be more specific (pause one minute). . . . Continue talking with your guide some more, asking her anything else you wish. (Pause one minute.)

It will soon be time to say goodbye to your guide for now. . . . Remember, she is always with you and you can come back to see her any time you wish. . . . Before you leave, ask your guide what you have to do *today* so that you will not have to eat compulsively (pause fifteen seconds). Make sure her answer is very specific (pause fifteen seconds). . . . When you are satisfied with her answer, make your goodbyes . . . and slowly come back to your existence here in the room and open your eyes.

Discussion of Guide

Do not be discouraged if you had difficulty with this fantasy. For those of you who have never tried a guided fantasy before, it may have been particularly difficult to relax or to visualize clearly. Like many new experiences, guided fantasies require you to master new skills. The more you practice, the better you will get at it. Yet even the most experienced of visualizers may have encountered difficulties with this fantasy. Let us deal with the most common problems separately.

1. "I couldn't find a guide."

    This is a common experience, especially for those new to fantasizing. I would suggest that you keep trying. Try the fantasy again, perhaps for several days in a row. Soon something will happen. Remember, not everyone actually sees her guide. You may just sense her presence or hear a voice in your mind. Sometimes, I find a woman will try too hard, so hard in fact that she is no longer relaxed. So just relax, be patient, and keep trying.

2. "My guide wouldn't talk to me."

    There could be several reasons for having difficulty in communicating with one's guide. Try asking your guide, "Am I not ready to hear what you have to say?" or, "Do I not *want* to hear what you have to say?" If your guide says "Yes," then ask her what you have to do to get ready to hear her. Often she will answer this type of question by saying, "You must continue meeting with me for some time before you can be ready to understand what I have to say."

    One of my patients, Paula, who had been working quite a while with her guide, reported during a group session that her guide had suddenly refused to communicate with her one day. I had her ask the guide why she was not talking, and having done so, Paula began to laugh. "She says I never listen to her anyway, and you know, she's right!" Paula suddenly realized that her guide had recently made several suggestions on how to handle a particular problem, all of which Paula had ignored.

3. "I don't understand my guide's answer."

    There are basically two explanations for such a difficulty.

More work may be needed to prepare yourself to deal with the meaning of the answer. In this case you might ask the guide how you can prepare yourself to understand her answer. Liala's experience will illustrate this process. During her fantasy her guide had given her a gift in answer to the question, "What do I need to do to allow me to give up my fat?" The gift she received was a picture of herself as a little girl, a picture of her skipping and playing. Though the meaning of such a gift may appear obvious to some, Liala had no idea what to make of her answer. I suggested she think about it during the week, and if by the following session Liala was still troubled by the image, we would work further with it. Liala set aside some time each day to talk with her guide and try to understand what her guide was trying to tell her, but by week's end she was still somewhat confused. So I had her imagine that she *was* that little girl in the picture, to envision herself as this person in the picture and imagine what her life was like as this little girl. Liala saw herself running and jumping and playing and filled with a joy of living that she had long forgotten. She saw her present self as an all-too-serious middle aged woman who had lost something dear to her: her joy. That joy, Liala realized, was what was missing from her life, and what she needed to recover in order to give up her fat. Another patient was told by her guide that in order to get over her compulsive eating problem she needed "peace and quiet." It took months of exploration and questioning of the guide to discover exactly that "peace and quiet" meant getting away from her husband, a move she had not been ready to make.

Another reason one might encounter difficulty in understanding the guide's responses is that the answers may not be clear enough or specific enough to be acted upon. Take, for example, the situation presented by Susan. She had been eating compulsively and asked her guide why. Her guide answered, "You need to relax." Such an answer, though it sounds reasonable, was too vague and general to provide guidance for her. Relaxing can range from napping, to taking up a sport, listening to music, practicing yoga, and so on. So I had Susan ask her guide, "What specifically do you mean by relaxing?" Another question which might help is, "What can I do right now, today, which constitutes relaxing?" One day the answer might be "lie down for half an hour," while the next it might be suggested you "go out for a run." Always try to get your guide to be as specific as possible.

Preface to Part of the Body You Do Not Like Fantasy

In this second guided fantasy, you will have the unique experience of talking with your own fat, trying to discover what it has to "say" to you and to the world. You will uncover some of the functions the fat may be serving. I suggest that you try this fantasy several times, each time using a different part of your body. You might find, as did one of my clients, that the fat on her thighs was "protecting" her genitals, while the fat on her upper back was helping her "shoulder a burden."

Part of the Body You Do Not Like . . .

Imagine yourself alone at home . . . no one is around and you will not be disturbed. . . . Spend a few minutes looking at yourself, nude, in front of a full length mirror. . . . Be aware of what you look like. . . . Try not to judge, just look. . . . See your face . . . your hair . . . your neck . . . your shoulders and arms. . . . Be aware of your chest . . . and your midriff . . . your waist. . . . See your hips . . . your thighs . . . your legs all the way down to your toes. . . . Turn a bit and see yourself from the back. . . . See your back . . . your backside . . . your legs. . . . Turn around again and face the mirror, and look at yourself a few moments. . . . Now, I would like you to focus on the part of your body which you dislike the most, the part where the fat upsets you the most. . . . If this part of your body had a voice, if it could talk, what would it say? (Pause twenty seconds.) . . . What message would it have for other people, the world? (Pause twenty seconds.) . . . What would the fat have to say to you? (Pause fifteen seconds.) Now, I would like you to imagine you *are* the fat (Pause ten seconds.) Imagine what it would feel like to *be* the fat on this person's body (Pause fifteen seconds.) What does the world look like from there? (Pause fifteen seconds.) What is your life like as this fat? (Pause fifteen seconds.) Become aware of the person to whom you are attached. . . . How does she feel about you? (Pause fifteen seconds.) How is she using you in her life? . . . What is she using you *for*? (Pause twenty seconds.) Are you able to do this for her? . . . In what way have you been her friend? (Pause thirty seconds.) Tell her how you feel. (Pause fifteen seconds.)

Now, become yourself again and look at yourself in the mirror . . . pay particular attention to the fat on the part of your body you do not like. . . . Does it look any different to you now? . . . Do you have any greater understanding of what it is doing for you now? Ask your fat how it would feel if you were to lose it. . . . Let the answer come from the fat. (Pause thirty seconds.) . . . And slowly come back to your existence here in the room and open your eyes.

Discussion of Part of the Body You Do Not Like Fantasy

Upon trying this fantasy, there are some who discover, much to their surprise, that the fat has been a friend to them. They have used the fat to help them out in ways they had never suspected. One woman, Janice, realized that she had been using her fat as a companion, a realization which came as somewhat of a shock to her. She had always experienced her fat as something negative, something destructive, and yet, through this fantasy, she discovered how her fat had indeed helped her deal with her loneliness. The thought of facing her lonely life without the fat actually frightened her. Of course, having realized the power she had been giving the fat—the power to stave off loneliness, to be a companion—Janice had taken but a first step. In order to lose the fat, she had to reclaim the power, to realize that fat is not, *cannot*, be a companion.

Another woman, Gert, chose her breasts as the part of the body she disliked most. She saw them as huge and cumbersome. Yet, after imagining herself to *be* these large breasts on her body, she became aware that she viewed them as making her appear matronly. They said to the world, "Here is a warm, motherly, caring person." When she asked her breasts what it would feel like if she were to lose some fat, they told her that she was afraid her personality would change: "I'm afraid that when I lose weight, people won't think I'm so nice anymore," she later told her group. It is important to realize that your fat is not a repository for your personality traits, and losing the fat does not mean losing a part of your personality that you cherish. Gert *was* a warm, motherly woman, and she liked being that way. Yet she discovered that she was viewing her warmth as a function of being fat. Just as Jennifer needed to "own" her sexuality, Gert had to "own" her warmth, to learn what it was about her that made her appear warm and empathetic to others. I asked Gert to spend some time observing her social interactions and to ask people she knew why they considered her to be warm and mothering. The responses surprised her. One woman told her it was Gert's eye contact and posture that made her feel Gert cared about what people were saying. Another man told her it was her smile, and another her bright eyes. Eventually, Gert came to realize that the warm, mothering part of her did not reside in her fat, in her large matronly looking breasts. It was only after this realization that she was able to lose weight without fear.

In analyzing your own experience with the fantasy, consider the following questions:

1. Which part of the body did you choose, and why did you choose *that* particular part to focus on? The fact that you chose to focus on your stomach instead of your thighs, for example, may have a significance. What special significance does this part have?
2. What messages did your fat seem to be sending out to the world? What was it letting them know about you? Is this the message you *want* to be sending? Your answer to this last question might be an immediate "no," but think a moment. Is it possible that your fat is saying something about you indirectly which you are afraid to state directly in words? For example, one of my patients, Barbara, had always been a "perfect little girl," always trying to live up to the standards of her demand-

ing, perfectionist parents. The one thing she held onto, the one area of her life she would not let them control, despite their disapproval of her weight, was her eating. Though she would not dare openly rebel against her parents, she held on to her fat as an indirect way of saying "See, I won't do or be everything you want me to be." Is *your* fat sending any indirect messages to the world? If so, what is keeping you from sending these messages more openly and effectively?

Preface to If My Fat Had a Voice

This fantasy deals with the relationship your fat has to other people in your life. It is most helpful to engage in this fantasy when you are aware that your fat is connected to someone in particular, but do not know in what way or what to do about it. Regardless of whether you are having difficulty with a particular individual, this fantasy can prove useful in uncovering connections your fat has to significant people in your life. You might want to use a parent, a lover or spouse, your child, a close friend, or a boss. There may be several people connected to your fat problem. Try this fantasy as many times as you wish, each time using a different person.

If My Fat Had a Voice

Imagine yourself to be in a room in which you feel comfortable. . . . Be aware of your surroundings . . . the furniture . . . the lights . . . the floors and walls. . . . Make sure it is a room in which you feel safe and comfortable. (Pause fifteen seconds.) . . . Now, imagine that the person you have chosen, the person to whom your fat is related in some way, is asking admittance to this room. . . . Let the person in, but place him or her wherever you desire, as near or far away as you wish. . . . See this person as clearly as possible. (Pause twenty seconds.) . . . See his/her clothes . . . hair . . . face . . . eyes. . . . How do you feel about having this person in the room with you? (Pause twenty seconds.)

Now, if your fat had a voice, what would it want to say to this person? (Pause fifteen seconds.) . . . Let the words come from the fat. (Pause twenty seconds.) . . . What is it trying to tell him/her? (Pause fifteen seconds.) . . . Continue talking with this person, but allow your responses to come out of the fat . . . let your fat talk. (Pause thirty seconds.)

Now, *become* this other person. . . . What does it feel like to be this person? (Pause twenty seconds.) . . . How is he/she viewing you? (Pause twenty seconds.) . . . How does he/she feel about your fat? (Pause twenty seconds.) . . . How does he/she view the whole situation? (Pause fifteen seconds.) . . . Become yourself again and look at the other person. . . . Do you have any greater understanding of him/her now? (Pause twenty seconds.) . . . Does your fat have anything more to say to this person? (Pause thirty seconds.)

Now, imgaine that all your fat has suddenly melted away. . . . You are still in the same room with this person. . . . Notice your positions in the room. . . . Have they changed? . . . Has *anything* changed? . . . Consider your relationship to this person now as a thin person. . . . How is it different? (Pause thirty seconds.) . . . What might the other person like about the change in you? (Pause twenty seconds.) . . . What might this person *not* like about this thin you? (Pause thirty seconds.) . . . How do you feel about this other person? . . . Are there any changes in the way you relate to him/her now that you are thin? (Pause thirty seconds.)

Now put the fat back on your body. . . . What more might it have to say to this other person now? (Pause twenty seconds.) . . . What is its message to this other person? (Pause fifteen seconds.) . . . When you are satisfied your fat has said all it wants to, slowly come back to your existence here in the room and open your eyes.

Discussion of If My Fat Had a Voice

Do not be discouraged if you had difficulty with this fantasy. Some people find it a particularly difficult one to do, especially at the beginning. Keep trying, though, and some rather surprising experiences may arise.

Most commonly the relationships explored in this fantasy are with a parent or spouse or lover. The experiences of some of my patients may illustrate the usefulness of such explorations.

Sometimes the fat provides a way of connecting to someone who is no longer living. Rebecca's fat was serving just such a function. She was a woman in her mid-fifties and had been in therapy with me for quite some time before discovering *any* functions her fat might be serving. So she was not expecting much when I announced to the group that we would be doing a guided fantasy aimed at uncovering the messages one's fat might have to a significant other, and how the fat is functioning in the relationship. Midway through the fantasy, however, I noticed she was crying, and her experience was so intense it became the focus of her therapy for months afterward. Rebecca had been orphaned at a very young age and had been reared by a woman she came to call "mother." Some years ago, her adoptive mother had also died. She insisted that though she loved her adoptive mother, she was very different from her in temperament, personality, and life style. In the fantasy, after letting the fat have its say, Rebecca realized that in her mind the fat had been a way of connecting up to her adoptive mother (who had been fat): "If I look like her, I'm her daughter." This realization shocked Rebecca and disturbed her for many months afterward. She feared that she would have to hold onto her fat forever in order to feel linked to her adoptive mother. It was some months later—when I asked her, "Do you have to look like someone to be her child?"—that she began to see that it was not necessary to look like her adoptive mother, not necessary to hold onto her fat, in order to feel she had really been her child. At that point, Rebecca was ready to take the power back from the fat and explore in what *other* ways she resembled her adoptive mother.

Sometimes the fat has a message for someone who is alive and involved in your life now, but to whom you are afraid to deliver the message directly. Dara began treatment some years ago as part of a group in which several of the women were dealing with the ways in which their fat entered into their marital relationships. It was clear to me, as it was to the other group members, that Dara's weight problem was tied up very closely with her husband, Jim, but she did not want to explore this issue, avoiding it whenever possible. One week we made a breakthrough, and Dara began opening up about her difficult relationship with Jim. For the next two weeks, she talked about Jim, his "old-fashioned background," and his expectations for her as his wife—expectations Dara could never meet. Apparently, he wanted a woman like his mother, who cooked large and lavish meals, cleaned, and met the needs of her husband selflessly. He was in ecstasy if he came home from work and found her on her hands and knees scrubbing the kitchen floor. The one similarity to his mother he did not want was a fat woman as a wife. He also wanted a wife to do her share of earning the family income. Dara worked a nightshift several times a week, came home, slept, and got up in time to do her chores and prepare him dinner. He was opposed to any outside help in caring for the house, though they could well afford it.

Upon hearing this oppressive situation, the group members began to support Dara enthusiastically, encouraging her to hire a housekeeper and tell her husband off. I realized that such support would be to no avail. If Dara had allowed herself to become involved in this situation, it must be serving some function for her to be treated this way. I suspected that her unhappy situation resulted from feelings of inadequacy and unworthiness. I saw that Dara was frightened by the encouragment of the others, and I feared she might avoid the issue by leaving the group. Not surprisingly, the following week she announced to the group that she was doing very well and had learned a lot from the group, enough so that she felt ready to leave and "try it out on my own." She said she was losing weight and was confident she would continue to do so after she left the group. Though she really believed what she was saying, I knew her leaving the group was an act of avoidance. Dara called me several months later and asked if she could see me individually. She had not lost any weight and had, in fact, gained considerably. She said she realized her problem with her weight was tied up to her relationship with her husband, and that she wanted to work with me on this connection. But when we got close to the real issues in their relationship Dara became frightened and left therapy.

A few months went by and I heard from Dara once more, though she made it clear that this time she was willing to explore how her problem with fat was tied up to her relationship with Jim, even if such explorations might lead to a divorce. From then on, we worked almost exclusively on how her marital difficulties were being manifested in her fat and her eating behavior. When, in the fantasy, she gave voice to her fat, it had some rather interesting things to tell Jim. One time it said, "I want to punish you. I'll take all you throw at me, but I'll get back at you by looking like this." In other words, her fat seemed to be her only source of rebellion. The fat sent another message to him as well: "I'm fat because you don't make me feel like a woman, a sexually desirable woman, so *I won't look like one!*" This message related to her dissatisfaction with their sexual relationship, a dissatisfaction which predated the development of her compulsive eating problem.

Let us take each message separately and explore how Dara was able to use the information obtained in the fantasy to take the power back from her fat.

Her fat's first message to her husband indicated that Dara was using her fat as a source of rebellion, a way of holding onto a piece of herself he could not control. In other words, she had given the fat the power to express her defiance. Realizing what power she had given the fat in this situation, Dara next explored *why* she had chosen to express the defiance through fat. She soon came to recognize the part she was playing in the relationship: "Everything that's happening to me is a result of how I'm thinking about myself. I haven't thought much of myself. Let's face it, I let him walk all over me." She had felt, on some level, deserving of his criticisms and unrealistic demands; yet a part of her struggled against accepting this view of herself. To defy her husband openly, to talk back, meant to upset the apple cart. She feared he would leave her. The only way Dara dared express the part of her that rebelled against his image (and her image) of herself was indirectly, through the fat. In order to take the power back from the fat, Dara had to learn to assert herself in the relationship, realizing she did indeed risk losing him, that he might not be able to adjust to the changes in her behavior. Interestingly, as Dara did begin to assert herself more, in ways she had practiced in our sessions, her self-image began to improve as well. As her self-image improved, she was less willing to put up with Jim's unrealistic demands. She even began to make demands of her own, and, as she was more able to openly express her objections, Dara's need to use the fat for defiance diminished. She had begun taking the power back from the fat.

As for the second message Dara's fat had for her husband, the sexual message, the process of taking the power back from the fat was a similar one, but in this case it was not necessary to resolve the problems in their sexual relationship. It was necessary only to disconnect the fat from the problem.

Dara had experienced difficulties in her sexual relationship with Jim from the start, yet somehow had forgotten about these earlier troubles. The focus of their arguments over sexuality during the past few years had been Dara's increasing obesity. Jim complained, "It's hard to make love to this fat woman. It's hard to get turned on when all I see is fat." Dara felt she had no right to make sexual demands on Jim, because of her "ugly body." She had given her fat the power to serve as the focus and as an excuse for her sexual frustrations and for Jim's lack of interest in her sexual pleasure. She did not want to take the power back from the fat, because to do so would be to face up to the fact that the fat was not the real cause of their problems. It was easier to hold onto the belief, "Some day our sexual relationship will improve. All I have to do is lose the fat." However, as Dara continued working with me, she slowly came to admit that there were some real sexual problems in her marriage and that these problems had existed well before she had become fat. It was important not only that she admit to herself that these problems existed, but that *they did not have to be resolved in order for her to lose the weight.* When she stated one day, "I'm facing the fact now that my sex life is not perfect, and it won't be perfect when I'm thin," it was clear she had finally disconnected the fat from the sexual problems in her relationship with Jim. She was now ready to give up the fat.

Dara's and Rebecca's experiences illustrate how the information obtained in this guided fantasy can be used to take the power back from the fat. I suggest that, in light of the messages your fat might have had for a significant person in your life, you consider the following questions:

1. Is the person someone involved in my life now or in the past?
2. Do I have any greater understanding now of how this person feels about my fat? Have I become aware of the part of this person that might actually want me to hold onto my fat?
3. Since the fat is only an indirect, imprecise way to convey my message, is there a more direct, effective way to let the person know what I have to say?
4. Am I afraid to state my message more directly and openly? If so, why? (Why did I give the power to the fat, and why don't I want to take it back?)
5. How can I learn to state my messages to this person without using the fat?
6. Is it necessary to resolve my conflicts with this person in order to give up my fat?
7. Am I using my fat as a link, a way to connect up to someone who is no longer a part of my life? If so, how can I retain what is or was valuable about this person without having to hold onto the fat?

These next few exercises are not guided fantasies, but like the previous fantasies, they aim at uncovering associations you have with "fat" and "thin." These associations can tell you a lot about the unconscious connections between your fat and your emotional state. In this first exercise, all you need to do is write down every word or phrase that enters your mind when you try to complete the sentence "I need my fat to. . . ." For example, you might write "I need my fat to . . . appear unattractive." Do not try to understand what you meant by "appear unattractive" or why those particular words came to mind—at least, not yet. Just write down *everything* you think of—without censoring, without judging or interpreting. At first you may have difficulty completing the sentence at all, but keep trying. Eventually the words will come. I need my fat to (or for):

Discussion of I Need My Fat

To illustrate how this exercise can be used to determine in what ways you may be using your fat, let us look at Dara's list. I need my fat to . . .

> relax
> keep people at bay
> suffer
> think I'm awful
> look disgusting
> appear unattractive
> stop competing with other women
> keep myself from looking good and helping Jim feel more like a man — he doesn't treat me like a woman. Why should I look good for him?

Dara looked over this list for a while and concluded that she was using her fat to meet several needs:

1. The need to relax. The first question I had asked Dara to consider was "In what way does fat allow me to relax?" Upon reflection, she discovered that when she imagined herself thin she also imagined herself in constant motion. In fact, her experience of being thin had been one of extreme activity. "I felt hyper," she said, as though, "now that I was thin, I had to be busy and involved in a lot of activities. I'd lost my excuse to stay home." Dara had many plans and expectations for herself when she was thin, "time to relax" not being among them. When fat, however, Dara thought poorly of herself, and her self-expectations were few. So when she needed to pull back a bit, to take a rest from accomplishing everything at once, Dara had to get fat.
2. Suffer, think I'm awful, look disgusting. On some level, Dara did not feel worthy of being thin, feeling good, and looking attractive. This feeling of unworthiness was evidenced in her list.
3. Stop competing with other women. When thin, Dara would often compare her body to other women's, and she did not like

the part of her that felt competitive with these women. Fat took her out of the arena of competition: "How can I even compete when I'm fat?"
4. Keep myself from looking good and helping Jim feel more like a man. In light of the earlier discussion of the functions of Dara's fat, it is not surprising to find that she needed to punish her husband. (It is interesting to note that using two different approaches aimed at uncovering the subconscious material — a sentence completion exercise as opposed to a guided fantasy — the same information can be obtained.)

Look over your own list now. See what more you can discover about how you are using your fat.

The following exercise is similar to the preceding one in that it requires you to complete a sentence with whatever comes to mind. It examines your association with "thin" as well as "fat," and will provide a good introduction to the next chapter. Include as many responses as you can think of. Again, do not attempt to censor or judge your responses. Write them down. The analysis will come later.

Fat is . . . .   Thin is . . . .

Discussion of Fat Is . . . . Thin Is . . . .

1. Do you see any patterns or themes among these words? Grouping similar words together in various combinations may help. For instance, on the "fat is . . ." list of Vickie, one of my patients, were:
    miserable
    sad
    a way of having troubles

    Vickie was very successful both financially and professionally. In fact, she felt *too* successful, as though she did not deserve all she had accomplished. So she held onto her fat as a "way of having troubles."

    Look again at your list. Can you change the order of some of

the words and phrases so that similar ones can be grouped together? What do these groupings tell you about yourself and the way you view your fat?
2. Are there any contradictions on your list? Some examples of contradictions found on others' lists:

    thin is . . . sexy   fat is . . . sick
          not sexy   healthy

What do the contradictions on your list tell you about yourself?
3. Are there any surprises on your list? Sometimes a word or phrase may appear on your list which surprises or even shocks you. One client was astonished to find "me" as a completion for "fat is . . ." Upon further exploration, it was discovered that she had been fat all her life and could not actually envision herself being any other way. As much as she desired a thin body, she identified herself in terms of a fat one. Not surprisingly, her "thin" list included "not me." Having discovered how closely her fat was tied to her sense of identity, she could then explore other components of her identity apart from the fat. ("What else makes me *me*?") She was able, after some time and much work, to envision herself thin and "still me." Another client was disturbed to see "death" appear on her list of associations with "thin." After discussing with her group the connections between death and being thin, she realized that the times she had been thin coincided with the death of significant people in her life. Thus she came to associate her being thin with the death of someone she loved. Though she realized this belief was irrational, she now feared the death of her children were she to lose weight once again.
4. Are there any discrepancies in length between your "fat is . . ." list and the "thin is . . ." list? Very often, the "thin" list is much longer, though the reverse may also be the case. What does this discrepancy tell you about your expectations and beliefs about "thinness" and "fatness"?
5. Are your two lists opposites of each other? In many cases, the "thin" list is all positive, and the "fat" list is all negative. If this is the case with your own lists, the discrepancy between the two can provide interesting information. It may indicate, for exam-

ple, that you view being thin as being in a state of constant happiness and perfection. Such an expectation is unrealistic and can lead to problems in maintaining a thin body once the weight has been lost. The next chapter will deal further with the expectations and beliefs you may have about life as a thin person.

The two lists can also be seen as representing two parts of the same person. For example, "self-hate" on the "fat" list and "self-love" on the "thin" list may indicate that a woman has formed her opinion of herself solely in terms of body weight, as though self-hate results only from being fat and being thin brings self-love. If she continues to view all her negative feelings about herself as stemming solely from her overweight, she will not be able to keep her weight down. Her image of herself as thin is one of feeling good about herself, with no room for ordinary feelings of self-doubt or self-hate. When she does become thin and encounters a situation which produces negative feelings about herself (losing a job or mishandling a social situation, for example) she will tend to put the weight on again. The bad feelings can then be attributed to excess weight, and she does not have to face what is really bothering her. Furthermore, getting fat would allow her to maintain the belief that "all I have to do to feel good about myself is lose weight."

The reality is that sometimes one may feel self-love and at other times self-hate or at least disappointment over not meeting one's standards or expectations. But such feelings must not become associated with one's body state. You can be thin and happy sometimes, and thin and unhappy at other times.

In light of the above discussion, consider your own list. See if you can take some of the emotions and descriptions that appear on your "fat" list, and envision yourself feeling and possessing those qualities *thin*. If "not sexy" or "unattractive" were on your "fat" list, for example, can you see yourself thin and feeling unattractive and not sexy? If the answer is no, then you have some rethinking to do. Believe it or not, there will be times after you get thin when you will not feel attractive or will not *want* to be seen as sexy (for instance, in a business situation). If thin means "sexy" to you, you will have to gain weight in order to feel "not sexy." Once you begin to disengage "attractiveness" and "sexiness" and "happiness" and "sadness" and so on from your body weight—once you begin to accept *all* aspects of your personality, negatives as well as positives, and integrate them into your self-image—you will be on your way to giving up your fat forever.

By now you have a clearer idea of how fat has been functioning in your life: what powers you have given to the fat. You have begun to take some of that power back and claim it as your own. You are ready to take the next step in your journey, to explore what being thin means to you.

three

The Reality of Thin

By now a clearer picture is emerging of what powers you have given to fat. Perhaps you have even begun to take some of that power back, and to disconnect the fat problem from the other problem areas in your life. This next leg of your inner journey will lead you to an exploration of "thin": what being thin means to you and why you might not be *letting* yourself become thin.

Your immediate reaction is likely to be something like, "Why *wouldn't* I want to get thin? That makes no sense. I've been fighting to get thin all my life." Susie Orbach often threw back another question when so confronted: "If being thin is so wonderful and desirable, how come you haven't gotten there in all this time or if you have, why did you gain it all back?" Why *haven't* you gotten thin? Think about that. Is it merely a lack of will power, a lack of character? Is it only because you love food so much?

The answer to these questions is complex—encompassing both emotional and physical factors. As we explored in the last chapter, you may not be losing weight because you need your fat to perform certain functions in your life. Or, you may not be able to get thin because you use food to meet emotional needs: you have given power to food just as you have given power to fat. "Emotional eating," not lack of willpower, may be keeping you from losing weight (this issue will be explored in chapter 6). Furthermore, you may begin to experience difficulty losing weight and maintaining the weight loss for physical reasons. Recent research studies have uncovered physiological problems associated with overweight and weight loss. We will explore this aspect of the problem in the final chapter. Finally, you may not be allowing yourself to become thin because of fears and fantasies about life as a thin person. Let us begin with the fears and unrealistic expectations you may hold about what it would be like to be thin.

What do you expect your life to be like when you grow thin? Whom will you be? Whom do you *expect* yourself to be? The answers to these questions are crucial to the determination of why you might still be holding onto your fat.

What do you expect your life to be like when you get thin? Your concept of life as a thin person has probably been shaped largely by the media. Thin women are happy, outgoing, sexy, bright, successful, " all together," even rich. Movies, commercials, television all convey this image. Think of your "thin is . . ." list from the preceding chapter. Does it reflect this image of thinness? The image is a myth. Thinness does not automatically bring with it happiness or success, nor do thin women have it "all together" by virtue of their body weight. The expectation that becoming thin will bring all these wonderful things into your life may be the very cause of your inability to lose weight permanently. I have heard women say, "I got thin and my husband didn't treat me any differently. My kids still left a mess for me to clean, and my job was just as boring," or, "When I got thin, men still weren't interested in me." It is very disappointing to discover that losing weight does not automatically guarantee a solution to your problems. In fact, many women regain their weight rather than face up to this discovery. That way, they can hold onto the belief that "Some day my life will be better (or I'll be happier, sexier, or more comfortable with men). All I have to do is lose weight." True, when you get thin there will be some positive changes in your life. You are likely to be more pleased with your appearance. You will have a wider selection of clothing. You may move and breathe more easily. Yet, if you are unhappy with yourself now, do not expect necessarily to be happy with yourself when you lose weight. Some of your self-displeasure may not stem from overweight alone. You may have a tendency to be disorganized or lazy or excessively shy and you may dislike these traits in yourself, but these traits will not disappear along with the weight. In order to avoid disappointment it is necessary to distinguish between your realistic and unrealistic expectations about life as a thin person. Several fantasies and exercises presented in this chapter will help you make such distinctions.

Often a woman will experience difficulty with thinness, because of her fears of whom she will be when thin. As we saw in the last chapter, some associate being thin with "not me." It is especially difficult for a woman who has been overweight all her life to envision herself thin. Being thin may be scary; it is an unknown. It can feel like a loss of identity. One of my patients, overweight since early childhood, lost fifty of her one hundred extra pounds while in her group. She left the group expecting to continue losing, but found herself stuck after losing only another ten pounds. For months her weight stayed the same. She came back to the group about six months later to work on why she could lose no more weight. It gradually became clear that all her life she had identified herself as a "fat woman." While she was losing weight she saw herself as a "fat woman in the process of getting thinner," but giving up these last forty pounds meant changing her identity to that of a "thin woman"—a step she was not yet ready to take. She needed time to prepare herself for this change in how she would define herself as a woman.

During a fantasy, another of my patients recalled a long-repressed incident that occurred after a large weight loss. Her husband passed her by on the street and "because I'd changed so much, he didn't recognize me. He didn't realize for a moment it was *me*." It was after this incident that she began putting back the weight "though I never made the connection until now. It's as though I wasn't *me* anymore."

Sometimes, the unease over who you will be when you get thin stems from a fear of what will be "let loose" by the loss of your weight. If you have given your fat the power to hold in certain desires, you may fear the loss of that fat, as though once the fat is no longer there, your hidden desires will take control of your behavior. As we discussed in the last chapter, fat does not "hold in" anything, so that a loss of fat lets nothing out.

There are women who have unrealistic expectations about who they *should* be when they get thin: "When I finally lose this weight

I'll be able to devote myself to developing a career." "When I get thin, I'll be more assertive. I won't let people push me around anymore." Such statements can lead to trouble. In the first instance, there is a belief that your weight is the only reason you are not succeeding in your career. Yet you might also fear there are other, less remediable factors involved. So you never let yourself get thin and put your belief to the test. In the second instance, if you are not assertive, if you lack the skills and experience necessary to get what you want, getting thin will bring no magic cure. Women tend to feel more confident when they are the "right size," but it is no easier to ask a man on the elevator to stop blowing cigar smoke in your face when you get thin. The assertive skills have to be learned. They do not come with a thin body.

Let us turn now to the fantasies and exercises which will help you become more aware of your own fears and expectations about life as a thin person. The first fantasy was derived from one developed by Susie Orbach, and its aim is to uncover some of your unconscious associations with thinness.[1] Before you begin, choose a social situation in which you were recently involved. Close your eyes and relax for a few minutes. Then begin the fantasy.

Thin Fantasy

Now review what happened in that situation. . . . Notice your clothes. . . . What were they saying about you? . . . How did you feel in your body? . . . How were you relating to the people around you? . . . Replay the scene as though you were viewing a movie in your mind. . . . Recall every detail.

Now, imagine yourself thin in that same situation. . . . What are you wearing now? . . . What are these clothes conveying about you? . . . How do you feel in your body? . . . Relive the situation, but this time as a thin person. . . . How might things have gone differently? (Pause one minute). . . . Do you feel more or less in control of the situation? (Pause thirty seconds) . . . Are people wanting or expecting different things from you? . . . Are you expecting different things from yourself? . . . Is there anything negative or frightening about being thin in this situation?

Discussion of Thin Fantasy

Reactions to this fantasy are often strong. "I had no idea I was expecting so much of myself when I got thin!" one woman was heard to say. "I expected a complete turnabout in my personality—as though I could handle anything that came my way by virtue of the fact that I was thin." Another woman, Sandy, had envisioned herself at a party she had attended the week before. Her experience at the party had been rather unpleasant. "I felt out of place and awkward. The other women were wealthy, sophisticated, well-educated and thin. When I saw myself at the party thin, nothing much was different. Sure I was thin and looked good, but basically I felt the same as before. The women were still wealthy, sophisticated and well-educated—things I feel I lack." Sandy's poor self-image clearly would not be mended merely by losing weight, yet she remarked, "I had thought that my only problem at that party was my weight. I'd thought to myself that night, 'If only I were thin, I'd feel comfortable here.' I can see now it just isn't so." A third woman who had also seen herself at a party envisioned herself surrounded by men—flirting, dancing, making passes at her. She had to leave the party in her fantasy because she did not know how to flirt, how to handle the passes; yet at the same time she wanted to reject these men, thinking, "Why do they suddenly want to pay attention to me now? Just because I'm thin? Where were they when I was a little heavier? It's only my body they want."

What did this fantasy reveal to you of your fears and expectations about being thin? The following questions will help you in analyzing your experience with the fantasy:

1. Was there a difference in the type of clothes you wore when you were fat and when you were thin? If so, how did your thin clothes differ? What was the message these clothes conveyed to the world? What were they saying about you? For example, they may have sent the message, "This woman is poised and attractive" or, "I am sexy" or, "I am a sophisticated woman." Do you feel comfortable with this message? Does it reflect who you *really* are or who you think you would like to be? One woman

wore short shorts and a tight red stretch tank top, with high heeled sandals. Though she had always thought she would like to dress in a sexy way when she got thin, in reality, the sort of outfit she had envisioned was not one she would *ever* feel comfortable in, fat or thin. She was surprised to learn that she did not really want to dress this way nor did she have to. Another woman, having envisioned herself in a similar sexy outfit, realized that while she might feel a little uncomfortable at first, such an outfit would express a part of her she wanted to develop.

2. How did you relate to others in the fantasy? Was the way you interacted with others purely a function of your weight or were there other factors involved? Realize that while it will be somewhat easier to deal with people thin in a world that has come to expect thinness from you, there are other aspects of your personality which enter into your interactions with others which will not change by virtue of your having lost weight. Take shyness, for example. You might claim, "I'll be less shy and self-conscious when I get thin, because I won't be so concerned with people's reactions to my weight." Yet, part of what makes you shy may have nothing to do with your weight. You may have developed a poor self-image apart from your weight, and you may not have developed the social skills needed for many social situations. If you believe that getting thin will eliminate all the parts of your personality you do not like you are letting yourself in for a disappointment, one that often leads to weight regained. It is a lot easier to stay fat and attribute your "faults" to the fat than to admit those "faults" are a part of you, fat or thin.

3. Were you able to get in touch with anything frightening about being thin? Though in the early stages women often claim there is nothing frightening or even negative about being thin, they may be harboring unrealized fears about who they will be or what they will have to face when they get thin. One woman in her early twenties, Linda, chose a situation for this fantasy in which she had had an argument with her father about going out. It was a beautiful spring day and he was prodding her to go out and enjoy herself. In her thin version, she felt more pres-

sure to go out. "When I'm thin I'll have no excuse to stay home. I bet he'll even expect me to got out with men. I might even feel I had to do it." Though Linda got in touch with fears of being thin, she remained afraid of going out, especially with men. Hence, she stayed fat.

Another way to get at your fears about being thin is to ask yourself the question: "What do thin women have to deal with that I don't?" The answer to this question will clue you into what frightens you, and what may be holding you back from getting thin.

The next fantasy further elucidates your fears and expectations about life as a thin person. It requires you to personify your fears or your needs to hold onto weight. In other words, you create a person in your mind who represents the part of you which will not let you get thin. It is not as hard as it sounds. Just try the fantasy and you will see what I mean.

Personification of the Part of You That Won't Let You Get Thin

Close your eyes and imagine yourself in a meadow at the edge of a forest. . . . It is a bright, sunny day. . . . Above you see the clear blue sky with little puffy white clouds. . . . Out in the meadow you can see wild flowers of many colors and shapes, with butterflies flitting from one to another. . . . Every now and then you can feel a gentle breeze on your face. . . . Spend a while relaxing and enjoying yourself in the meadow. (Pause one minute.)

Now, look toward the forest, and you will notice a path leading deep into the woods. . . . Far away, at the end of the path, a figure is coming toward you. . . . You cannot see her clearly yet, but you know that she is the personification of the part of you that will not let you get thin. (Pause twenty seconds.) . . . As she approaches you, you begin to see her more clearly . . . her face . . . her hair . . . her eyes . . . her body . . . the clothes she wears. . . . As she approaches you, she tells you that she is a messenger from your subconscious and that she is here to tell you why you hold onto your weight, why you will not let yourself get thin. . . . Walk with her a bit at the edge of the forest. (Pause twenty seconds.) . . . Find a comfortable spot under a tree and sit down. (Pause twenty seconds.) . . . Now she is going to tell you why you are holding onto your weight, why you have not been able to get thin. Take a few minutes to listen and then you can ask her questions about what she said. (Pause three minutes.) . . . Ask her if there is any way to work out a compromise, so that her needs could be met as well as your needs to lose the weight. (Pause two minutes.) Prepare to say goodbye to her for now. (Pause twenty seconds.) . . . She gets up and begins to walk back down the path, then she turns back to you and hands you a gift — something which will help you to give up your weight. (Pause twenty seconds.) . . . Look at what she gave you. See if you can discover the significance of this gift. (Pause twenty seconds.) . . . She continues on down the path, and you walk back into the meadow. . . . Lie down and relax and give yourself some time to absorb the experience you have just had. (Pause thirty seconds.) . . . And whenever you feel ready, come back to your existence here in the room and open your eyes.

Discussion of Personification Fantasy

The versatility and intensity of this fantasy make it an invaluable one in your search for insight into your weight problem. In addition, it may provide you with some direction or even explicit instructions as to how you can get thin. The fantasy will show up again, in slightly altered form in the final chapter of the book.

Let us begin our discussion of the fantasy with an examination of some of the experiences of others. One woman, Allison, discovered two reasons for not getting thin which were exerting a powerful influence on her behavior, both of which she was unaware of until she tried the fantasy. She first discovered that she was unable even to attempt getting thin because of a fear of failure. "I've failed so many times before, on so many diets. Even when I was able to lose weight I'd quickly gain it back. Each time I was successful I'd think, 'This is it. This diet really works, I'm thin forever.' " But, with each weight gain and subsequent disillusionment came an increasing sense of distrust and self-loathing. It was no wonder Allison was afraid to commit herself. What if she were wrong, what if she failed again? It was easier not even to try losing weight.

Our work together was three-fold. First, I made it clear to Allison that there is no success or failure in this approach to the eating problem. It is not a *program* to be followed to the letter, but rather a way of thinking about and working on your compulsive eating problem. Weight loss is not an absolute, immediate goal. You cannot fail with this method. *Any* changes you make in your eating and your weight and your self-image are positive improvements. If Allison was not ready to lose weight now or next week or even next year, that would be okay. Second, I tried to clarify for Allison the difference between her experience of losing weight in the past and what it would be like to lose weight now. In the past she just dieted, paying little or no attention to her emotional needs or the psychological ramifications of losing weight. Her approach to weight loss would be radically different this time, as she worked through the reasons she got fat in the first place, as she took the power back from the fat, as she no longer used food to meet emotional needs, and as she explored her hidden fears about thinness. Allison would lose weight because she had changed—in her relationship to food, to fat, to her whole self—not because she had temporarily imposed a diet on herself. Finally, we worked on the issue of trust in herself. Allison had no reason to trust herself with respect to food and dieting. She had failed so many times before. However, as she progressed in the group and began to understand *why* she did what she did and how she could change, Allison became less judgmental and more accepting of herself. Allison began slowly to trust that she knew how to take care of herself: how to calm herself down without food, how to protect herself without a buffer of fat.

This fear of failure is a common one in women who have tried repeatedly to get thin. Another common fear, which was Allison's second discovery from her fantasy, equates thinness with perfection or with pressure to accomplish. "If I get thin I'll be perfect, and I can't deal with that"—or, as in Allison's case, "If I get thin, if I've finally accomplished this life-long task, then I'll have to go on to change in other ways as well. I'll have to go on to improve in all the other ways I've been putting off." It's as though concentration on getting thin has allowed Allison to put aside other self-improvements. When she gets thin, she will then expect herself to begin tackling these other problem areas—lack of assertiveness, procrastination, lack of exercise—a prospect that seemed overwhelming. Again, it is easy to see why Allison might not be letting herself get thin: there's so much more she will expect of herself as a thin person. Allison's work was to separate her hopes and expectations from her bodily states. Allison could choose to work on her problem with assertiveness now, at her present weight, or she could decide she was not ready to deal with this issue, and promise herself that even if she got thin she did not have to resolve or even begin working on assertiveness. Such an approach aims at separating the issue of getting thin from other issues in your life. It allows you to get thin without any strings attached.

It is important to clarify Allison's situation at this point. Remember that prior to doing the fantasy Allison was basically unaware of why she was not able to get thin. It was through the experience of the fantasy and much subsequent thought and analysis that she became aware of the fears and expectations she had associated with being thin. In analyzing your experience with the fantasy consider the following questions:

1. What image did your personification take?

Every woman who tries this fantasy has her own unique personification, a reflection of her inner fears and expectations about losing weight. You were asked to get in touch with that part of you that will not let you get thin and to give that part of you a body, a form. The resulting personification is a personal symbol from your subconscious. It can tell you something.

One woman saw her personification as a midget, the message being that there was very little left that was keeping her from getting thin. Another patient's image was of a cartoon character, Veronica, from the Archie comic strip. This image represented the part of her that holds onto a fantasy of what she always wanted to look like. On some level, she knows she will never look the way she wants to look, even when she gets thin, but she holds onto the fantasy by staying fat. That way she can still believe that some day she will look just the way she had always dreamed—all she has to do is lose fifty pounds. The image was trying to tell her that her hopes were indeed fantasy—hence, the cartoon character. In order to lose the weight she would have to face the reality that nothing, not even weight loss, would make her look as she had always desired.

Another woman, Kathy, saw her personification split in two —one half a sophisticate, the other half a "tramp," swinging her pocketbook. This image was a clue to Kathy's fears about being thin. She expected to be both a sophisticate and a tramp. She had little difficulty accepting the sophisticate, but was horrified by the image of herself as a "tramp." Further exploration revealed that in her teen-age years she had, in fact, been thin and wore provocative, sexy clothing. Her father had often called her a tramp. In her mind, there was a close association between thinness and sexual promiscuity. In order to allow herself to get thin, she had to explore her fears and conflicts about expressing her sexuality and to learn that it is okay to express one's sexuality through dress—at any weight.

At another time, Kathy imagined a very different personification, but one which stemmed from another part of her that would not let her give up the weight. The image was one of herself thin, dressed in a ballet outfit. This image represented the part of her that had always expressed her creativity through dance, a part she had lost many years before. She had been an excellent ballerina, encouraged by her teachers to continue professionally, but just at the height of her success Kathy's mother began sabotaging her efforts to continue and Kathy was forced to give up her dancing. At various points in her life, Kathy felt her mother had attempted to sabotage Kathy's success. Even now, as an adult, she feared her mother would attempt to sabotage her success once again. Of course, Kathy had much to explore and work through after this realization, but it was at least a first step, providing her with a direction in which to work. Without the conscious knowledge of her fears of thinness, Kathy would not have been able to lose weight permanently.

Finally, another image, which in itself conveyed a message, was Sandy's personification in the form of a glass figure, which represented her fear that as a thin woman she would be fragile and unprotected. She viewed her fat as providing cushioning for a fragile, sensitive self.

What does your own choice of image tell you? What was your subconscious mind trying to convey to you through its choice of images?

2. What did your personification tell you in words?

Much of this fantasy dealt with direct, verbal messages from your personification as to why you have not been letting yourself grow thin. The following examples may help you in analyzing your own fantasy. One woman, Michelle, discovered a fear of getting thin which surprised her. Her personification told her that she feared, "If I let go of the fat, the whole world will know who I really am." She felt on a deep level that the core of her was "bad," and, "If I take away the fat, everyone will see it." The work in such a case was twofold: exploring Michelle's poor self-concept that fat did not do anything for Michelle. If she felt covered and hidden by the fat, it is because *she had given the fat the power to hide her "true" self.* Conversely, giving up the fat does not mean losing protection. This concept is an important one and we shall return to it later in the chapter.

In another instance, Jackie's personification represented a part of her that would be abolished if she were to get thin. It represented her warmth and caring and sensitivity. When she explored further, Jackie revealed a distrust of and dislike for thin people. She could not think of any thin people she did not consider self-centered or insensitive. Were she to lose weight, she feared she would become like them. Her work consisted in exploring her perception of thin people and her fears that *she* was selfish and insensitive and was covering that part over with fat. Another woman, whose personification also represented a part of her she feared would be abolished when she gave up the weight, had another solution. Her personification told her that it was not necessary to abolish the trait, but to integrate it into her perception of herself. The woman pictured herself absorbing the personification into her being.

Finally, another patient, Betty, saw the personification as

herself as a little girl. She told Betty, "I'm the one you haven't let go of yet. You've never made peace with your past." Betty realized that "Until I am ready to make peace with my childhood, this little girl will hang onto my hips." What exactly constituted "making peace" with her childhood was the subject of many sessions thereafter, but the important point is that through this fantasy, Betty became aware of previously unconscious obstacles to giving up the weight. Again, the understanding gained from the fantasy gave her a direction in which to work.

Similarly, your own personification told you something which will help you uncover the reasons that you have not been letting yourself get thin, though the meaning of what it said may not be immediately clear. Take some time to consider what it said.

3. What was the significance of the gift she gave you?

Just as the image your subconscious chose to represent the part of you that will not let you get thin has significance, so does the gift the personification gave to you. The gift was given as "something which will help you give up your weight," so no matter how cryptic the message, your subconscious mind is telling you something with its choice of gifts. Let us look first at some of the gifts others have received.

One woman who had discovered she needed to be more accepting of herself—both her positive and negative traits—in order to get thin, received a mirror, with the message "the only place you are going to get the acceptance you need, is from yourself." Another received a pitchfork, signifying "It's time to get to work." A third was given a tiny gold fork, emphasizing her need to make each meal important, with careful attention to her eating: taking small bites and enjoying each one. One woman, who had discovered from the fantasy that she feared being thin because she would feel weak and powerless, received a check for an exercise class which emphasized working out with weights. Another woman, who was about to leave the group to go away to school, was given a box filled with gold coins. Each coin was a memory, and whenever she was feeling lonely in her new home, she could look at the coins. She was also given a scroll to fill up with the events of her new life. She was to write down each incident that occurred, and it would become a coin and enter the box. Finally, a woman who had learned from her personification that there was no longer anything keeping her from getting thin got a hug and a kiss goodbye.

What was the the message of your own gift? If you are still having difficulty discerning the message, think about the gift in relation to what the personification has said to you. From the above examples, it is clear that the gift usually relates to what the personification said about why you are not able to get thin. Since the gift's purpose is to help you in being able to give up the weight, its meaning will become apparent if you relate it to these earlier messages.

You can also ask yourself, "What is the function of the object I was given?" What words are usually associated with the object? For example, in the case where the woman was presented with a pitchfork, the thinking might have gone as follows: "My personification told me that I wasn't taking my work here in the group seriously enough — that in order to get thin, I'd have a lot more work to do. The gift she gave me was a pitchfork. What associations do I have with that word? . . . 'the devil'. . . . No, that doesn't fit . . . 'work' . . . maybe she was telling me, it's time to dig in and get to work. . . . Yes, that feels right." Sometimes you may not be pleased with the message implied by the gift, as was the case in the above example, but the message is important, nonetheless.

The next fantasy will give you more insight into your fears and expectations about life as a thin person.

Visualization of Self in a Thin Body

Relax and close your eyes. . . . Imagine yourelf in a bright sunny room. . . . As you look around, you see beautiful potted plants, and fresh flowers on a table. . . . Soothing, peaceful music fills the air. . . . Spend a few minutes just relaxing and enjoying the warmth of the sun as it streams through the window. (Pause thirty seconds.) . . . The window is slightly open and a cool, refreshing breeze enters the room. . . . Breathe deeply and allow yourself to relax in this beautiful room. (Pause one minute)

This room is a very special, magic place. . . . You are in a place which will provide you with the unique opportunity of briefly experiencing what it would be like to live within another's body. . . . Lining the walls are black bound books containing pictures of thousands of people. . . . Walk over to the row of books marked "Thin Women" and take down one of the books. . . . As you turn the pages you see pictures of many thin women. . . . Some are famous actresses or movie stars, some models, some may be cartoon characters. . . . There are political figures and "sex symbols." . . . You may even find pictures of women you know . . . friends, relatives who are thin. . . . Flip through the pages for a few minutes until you come to one woman whose body you would like to try on. (Pause one minute.) . . . There may be more than one body you would like to try, but just for now, pick one. . . . Once the choice has been made, you have only to insert the picture in the slot next to the bookcase. (Pause fifteen seconds.) . . . Now, you will notice a door opening to the left of the slot. . . . Walk through the door and when you emerge on the other side, you will find yourself in the body of the person you have chosen. (Pause thirty seconds.) . . . How does it feel to be inside this body? (Pause twenty seconds.) Do you feel lighter, quicker, sexier, less protected, weaker? Find your own words to describe the feeling of moving around in this thin body. (Pause one minute.) . . . Would your life be any different now were you to live in this body? If so, in what way? (Pause thirty seconds.) . . . Spend a few minutes more checking out all your reactions, positive and negative, to living in this other woman's body. (Pause one minute.) . . . When you feel ready, step through the door into the room and back into your own body. (Pause thirty seconds.) . . . It will soon be time to leave this special room for now, but remember, you can come back as often as you wish. . . . Slowly leave the room and your fantasy and open your eyes.

Some women are surprised to find that they did not feel comfortable in another's body. One woman discovered that "I want to keep my own body." Another found the burden of living in a "sexy" body overwhelming. "I didn't want to always be seen as sexy, but in Sophia Loren's body, it seemed impossible not to be so."

For the next exercise, it is necessary only to make a list of all the things you are putting off doing until you get thin.[1] It may take some thought, but I am sure there are many things you will not do or experience, because you are not yet thin. "Buying clothes" is a common example. Do not judge or analyze your responses. For now, I just want you to list everything you think you are denying yourself or will not do or buy until you get thin.

List of Everything I'm Putting Off Doing Until I Get Thin

Some of you may have had long lists. How sad to think that we are denying ourselves pleasures of life just because we have more fat on our bodies than our culture and society (or we ourselves) think we ought to have. Let us look at the experience of one of my patients, Audrey. Despite many changes in her eating behavior and her awareness about the functions fat was playing in her life, she was unable to lose any weight. I suggested filling out the list. Her list covered an entire page and included:

    buying new clothes   taking up cooking
    going back to school   exercising

Let us take each item from her list and examine it separately:

Buying new clothes: This item is likely to have appeared on many lists. Women most often deny themselves the pleasure of wearing clothing in which they feel comfortable and attractive because they are fat or because they feel they are going to lose weight. Unfortunately, such women can put off buying themselves clothes indefinitely. When I was eating compulsively, I was forever planning diets which would take off my unwanted weight "forever." I would put off buying myself new clothes until I lost the weight—again and again. Such was the case with Audrey, too. Year after year she denied herself the pleasure of new clothing. As you will learn in the next chapter, clothing conveys messages to the world about who you are, and you are just as entitled as any thin person to choose those messages carefully. As Audrey explored her feelings about clothes, she came to feel it was okay to begin buying herself comfortable, attractive clothing to fit her body *now*. She came to view buying new clothing as a self-affirmation and a sign that she was beginning to accept herself just as she was.

Going back to school: The first questions that came to mind when I saw this item on Audrey's list were, "Does she really want to go back to school? Is she ambivalent? Or does she think if she got thin she should or would have to go back to school?" Further exploration revealed that Audrey did indeed want to go back to school, but feared that she would feel too self-conscious about her body to relax in class. In reality, Audrey was not very much overweight — perhaps twenty pounds over her "ideal" — yet in her own mind she experienced herself as huge, and she felt she would stand out in the classroom. Part of her work consisted in adjusting her body image to be more in line with reality, but she also needed to explore her fears about standing out, being different. Beginning to catch on, Audrey exclaimed one day, "Why should I deny myself an education just because I have some extra pounds of fat on my body? If the other students don't like me, that's their problem!" Audrey's new way of thinking would be as valid, by the way, for a woman seventy pounds overweight.

Taking up cooking: Audrey had long been interested in exotic and tasty recipes from all over the world, and had amassed quite a collection. However, she kept putting off trying them out until she got thin, thinking, "A fat woman shouldn't eat those foods. Fat women should be on diets." Unfortunately, Audrey had been denying herself the pleasure of cooking and eating those dishes for many years — always putting off the cooking until she finished her diet. But Audrey was always on a diet! As you will see in the chapter on eating awareness, there is no reason, barring medical restrictions, to deny yourself any foods you desire. Extra body weight can be lost without dieting and without self-denial. In fact, as Audrey began allowing herself to cook and taste delicious foods she found herself eating less. She got so much enjoyment from these foods, it took much less to satisfy her. The long years of denial of pleasurable eating experiences had led, at least in part, to the huge eating binges and subsequent weight gains.

Exercising: Again the question arose: Did Audrey really want to

The Reality of Thin 75

begin exercising or was she using her fat as an excuse not to do something she really did not *want* to do? In this case, Audrey's response was unclear and reflected her ambivalence. On the one hand, she felt that a thin body would move more freely and easily. In part, there is some validity to her belief. It is easier to move a body with no extra fat on it. However, I have seen women who are substantially overweight develop the grace, skill, and agility of highly trained athletes and dancers. Let us not forget that Isadora Duncan was overweight, even by the standard of her day, and yet she was considered one of the most graceful dancers of all time. One of my patients, 5'2" and 160 pounds, took up belly dancing and became so proficient that she was able to become a teacher.

On the other hand, Audrey was not sure she wanted to exercise. Further examination of her feelings revealed a belief that she *should* begin exercising, and she felt she would have to do so when she got thin. After exploring this "should" some more, Audrey discarded her belief, and promised herself that she would not have to take up exercising, fat or thin, unless she began to feel a real desire to do so.

Audrey went through her entire list, separating out what she did not want to do from that which she did desire but had been denying herself because of her fat. Then she systematically set out to do all those things she had always wanted to, regardless of what anyone thought of her. She bought new clothes, applied to graduate school, took a Chinese cooking class, even decided to take up running the following spring. During this time her weight dropped slowly, but steadily. She was no longer waiting until she got thin to enjoy her life.

In analyzing your own list, the following questions may be helpful. Look over each item when considering a question:

1. Is the item some pleasure you have been denying yourself just because you are not thin? If so, perhaps it is time to give up your old beliefs about what you should or should not do when you are fat. It might be easy for some of you to look at a woman like Audrey who is only slightly overweight and think, "She wasn't so fat, I don't know why she thought she couldn't buy clothes or go to school." It does not matter that the world did

not consider Audrey obese. She considered herself fat and undeserving, and denied herself pleasure based on those beliefs. No matter how overweight you are, you are probably doing the same thing to yourself. Look over your list again. How many of those items could you really be doing now?

2. Is the item a reflection of what you feel you "should" do when you get thin?

   Audrey's inclusion of exercising on a list of things she is putting off until she gets thin was an example of such an item. In actuality she was putting off exercising because she really was not sure she wanted to exercise at all. Being overweight was providing her with an excuse not to do something she felt she "should" do.

3. Why are you not doing the things on your list? Is the fact that you are not yet thin actually keeping you from doing what you want?

   This question is a combination of the first two. It requires that you think about each item and discover the real reasons you are not doing it. Again, all that may be keeping you from doing what you want, from enjoying your life more fully, is your belief about what fat people can or cannot, should or should not do. Maybe it is time to start enjoying the things you like to do, no matter what other people think.

   Enjoying your life now, and no longer waiting until you get thin to start living, will not only make for an immeasurably happier life, but will also make it easier for you to lose weight. Being thin will lose some of its specialness and magic, because you will have already stolen and adopted into your life some of its supposed benefits. At the same time, your concept of what life as a thin woman would be like will be based on reality. You will have already incorporated your concept of what thin women do into your own lifestyle. You will have begun building a new identity separate from your body weight.

Self-identity is the subject of the final exercise of this chapter.[2] The exercise requires another list which might prove a challenge.

Distinctive Qualities

What is it that makes you "you"? What is it that distinguishes you from other people? What makes you unique? It may not be any one particular quality but a combination of many qualities. Make a list of those qualities which identify you as you:

As we have seen, fat may become a part of a woman's identity, to the point where she defines herself primarily in terms of her fat—as though all there was to her was fat. Either she ignores or disregards her other traits or she connects her fat with those traits, as though they resided within the fat. Take the example of the woman who considered herself warm and caring, but who feared that when she got thin she would become insensitive and self-centered.

The list you have just completed will help you to discover those qualities you possess which are distinctive to you, which identify you as "you." I hope that in your analysis of the list you will discover that those qualities are a part of you, no matter what your weight, and you will be able to incorporate them into your self-identity. Therefore, when you get thin, you will fear losing nothing but your fat.

Let us look at Natalie's list. Her experience may help elucidate your own.

good voice	procrastinator
efficiency	escapist
fast working	fearful
ability to reorganize a situation and handle it	good hostess, cook, and decorative table setter

My first reaction upon reading Natalie's list was that she had left out those qualities I most associated with her: quick wit, extremely intelligent, with a zest for cultural pleasures in life—a zest she conveys to others, sparking their own interest. Other members of her group confirmed my perceptions. Why had Natalie omitted her most distinctive and likeable qualities? In part, she was not really aware that others perceived her this way. However, upon further reflection, she came to realize that her list reflected those qualities her husband both valued and criticized. Her husband might just as easily have drawn up the list. Natalie's perceptions of herself were so much those of her husband that she used his criteria to judge herself, rather than her own sense of who she was. In fact, other than her husband's (and before that her father's) judgments about her, Natalie had no sense of self.

Carrie's list reflects another aspect of the problem. She included the following qualities:

intelligent	articulate
moody	organized
sensitive	pretty
not athletic enough	warm

Her list appeared to be a fairly accurate representation of herself, yet she had difficulty owning some of these qualities as parts of herself, separate from the fat. I had asked her, "Which of these qualities you have listed do you know you will take with you when you get thin?" Some of the traits—intelligent, articulate, pretty—gave her no trouble, but others, such as "sensitive," proved difficult to separate from her perception of herself as fat. Feeling she had developed her fine sensitivity because of the hurts she had experienced as a fat woman, Carrie feared that this hard won trait she admired in herself would be lost when she got thin. She viewed thin people as insensitive and self-centered, and could cite numerous examples of such people. Furthermore, she feared that as she became thin and more self-centered, she would have less energy to give to other people.

It was easy to see why Carrie was unable to get thin. At least on some level, she feared getting thin, because she believed that to do so would mean giving up part of her identity—a part she cherished. Our work after that consisted in exploring what Carrie meant by "self-centered." Did focusing on herself preclude caring for others? She explored fears she had about finding out she was a truly self-centered, insensitive person, and like Jackie, the woman we met earlier in the chapter, that she was covering this part of her up with fat. She examined her belief that there was something wrong with focusing on her own needs rather than others, at least *some* of the time. Carrie's idea of being warm, caring, and sensitive meant that she be available to help others *at all times*, regardless of her own needs. As she came to change her views on what constitutes "self-centeredness" she also came to see that focusing on oneself and satisfying one's needs does not, in fact, preclude caring about others. Furthermore, getting thin need not mean giving up any traits, any qualities—anything—save the fat.

In analyzing your experience, keep the following questions in mind:

1. Which of these qualities will you take with you when you get thin?

    The answer to this question ought to be, in most cases, "all." Personal qualities do not disappear when you get thin, and even those qualities which appear totally connected with fat will still remain to some extent when you get thin. For example, let us say that "shy" or "self-conscious" appeared on your list. It could be argued that you feel shy or self-conscious because of your overweight, fearing the disapproval of others; yet think for a moment. Is your shyness *entirely* a result of your fat? If you were fat as a child, you may have become shy and self-conscious as a result; yet the fact remains that you *are* shy and self-conscious and have never learned to feel comfortable in social situations. Certain social skills that people learn to help them along in social situations are lacking. Getting thin will not make the discomfort go away completely. For those of you who became fat later in life, ask yourself, "Was I ever shy or self-conscious (or any trait you attribute to your weight) before I got fat?" Very likely the answer is "yes."

    Let me use my own personal experience to illustrate this point. My own list would have included both "shy" and "self-conscious." I would have stated that my difficulty in attending social functions was directly related to my fat. "If only I were thin, I'd feel comfortable—a part of things," I used to say to myself. Yet getting thin did not alleviate my discomfort significantly. Yes, I felt secure in the knowledge that I looked attractive, but basically I was still shy and self-conscious. I still sat in the corner of the room, afraid to talk. All my life I had been shy and had therefore not learned the social skills necessary to function with ease in social situations. Furthermore, despite my new "thin" body, I still felt self-conscious. The reality was that I felt uncomfortable with my body, period. Much work needed to be done to allow me to feel comfortable with my body, at any weight.

2. Which of these qualities do you fear you will not be able to take with you when you get thin?

Like Carrie, you may see certain characteristics of yourself you admire or even cherish as tied only to your fat. If so, what makes you think these qualities are dependent on your fat? Can you learn to separate them and own them as parts of you separate from your bodily state? Can you promise yourself to take those traits with you?

3. What qualities did you omit from your list?

Much can be learned from what you did not remember or did not think of putting on the list, as we saw in Natalie's case. One way to discover what you left out is to put the list away for a few days or weeks and then look at it again. Is there any trait that strikes you by its absence? Or you could ask others to give you a list of their perceptions as to what makes you "you," or have them look over your own list to see if they notice any conspicuous omissions.

Merely sitting down and thinking out the list will have been of help to many of you. You might discover that, as one woman put it, "I defined myself! I am really a person. It had nothing to do with the fat!" The closer you can come to defining yourself apart from the fat, the closer you will come to being able to get thin.

I hope this chapter has helped you become aware of some of your fears and unrealistic expectations about being thin. The next chapter will help you further in losing the weight by focusing on your body, how you feel about it, and preparing you to live in a thinner body.

four

Bodywork

"I don't experience myself from the neck down."

"I can't stand to look at myself in a mirror."

"Sometimes I feel so fat; other times I feel thin—and I can feel both fat and thin in a single day!"

"Sometimes when I look in the mirror I don't know who that person is looking back."

Do any of these statements sound familiar? Statements such as these are made every day in my office. They reflect distorted and unclear body images and are characteristic of women with all kinds of eating problems—from anorexia to bulimia and obesity. Women with eating disorders are notorious for having distorted body images, viewing themselves as either fatter or thinner than they actually are. Such problems complicate efforts to get thin. It is the purpose of this chapter to help you explore your body concepts and make you more aware of your body. Such awareness is essential for a woman who wants to be able to lose weight permanently or to get over an eating problem.

First, what is meant by body image or body concept? It is your sense of possessing a body with clear boundaries separating yourself from the rest of the world. It is your awareness of how much space you take up in the world, a realistic sense of how large or small you are in relation to people and things around you. It is your awareness of the body's parts and your sense of control over them.

The most comprehensive definition of body image or identity

which I have encountered is found in Hilde Bruch's *Eating Disorders*. Her definition includes:

1. The correctness in perceiving and identifying internal body signals (for instance, the ability to distinguish the stomach rumblings of hunger from the stomach upset of nervous tension).
2. The accuracy with which one distinguishes between internal bodily signals and external (outside) stimuli.
3. The sense of control and ownership of one's bodily functions.
4. The attitude toward one's body structure. Some aspects of your body makeup are structural and cannot be changed—broad shoulders, heavy thighs in proportion to torso, height, and so on. The attitude toward these body structures can be positive or negative depending on cultural preferences and what an individual has been taught about her body.[1]

For the most part, women in our culture who have eating problems have poorly developed body concepts—they are "out of touch" with their bodies, and the awareness of body they do possess is reflected in negative attitudes. Why is this so? How a woman feels about her body is very much a function of what others have taught her. In some cultures, large hips and breasts are valued as signs of fecundity and beauty. A woman possessing such qualities would be praised as beautiful and desirable, and thus she would have developed a positive body image, viewing her body as pleasurable and desirable. Yet the same woman in another culture (ours for example) would quickly learn that her large breasts and broad hips are undesirable and her body image would likely reflect such negative attitudes. She would experience her body as gross, ugly, and unacceptable.

Such differences in the way a young woman views her body are not only cultural. Fashionable weights change almost yearly within a culture, and what was considered an acceptable body one year may be rejected the next. I think of the many of you reading this book who thirty years ago would have found your present weights acceptable, but who in this era of extreme thinness feel the need to diet your bodies down to new lows. You may spend countless hours thinking about diets and food, depriving yourselves constantly; yet had the standard of beauty remained as it was during Marilyn Monroe's time, you would be pleased with your body right now. How much time and self-hatred has gone into trying to fit our bodies to an unrealistically thin standard?

Since so few of us have "ideal" bodies, most of us have to some degree a negative body concept. We dislike our hips or thighs or backsides or other body parts which do not fit our image of what is right or desirable. For those of us who were heavy since birth or early childhood, or who, as girls, possessed bodies with unusual proportions (short, heavy legs or large stomachs, for example), the problem is even greater since we have had to deal not only with general cultural values, but with very specific negative feedback from others—sometimes even from the ones we loved and depended on in forming our concept of "self." These negative judgments would have a potent effect on one's developing body concept.

Perhaps these negative body images we have formed underlie, in part, the unclear body concepts women with eating problems exhibit. As the statements at the beginning of this chapter indicated, such women are often "out of touch" with their bodies. It is understandable that if a woman judges her body negatively, then she would want to reject that body, cut off her awareness of it, and such is often the case. "I hate my body. I don't want to feel it. I don't want to be reminded of it," one woman explained, and so she saw herself as residing totally in her head. "I don't experience myself from the neck down." She viewed everything below her head as an undifferentiated mass, with which she would rather not be associated.

Ironically, on one level, this woman was extremely aware of her body, in her self-consciousness and discomfort about others' reactions to her size; yet she still did not really "feel" her body, experience it. Her self-consciousness and awareness of her fat was merely a concept in her head, not a felt sense of her fat. In her mind she knew she was fat, but she rejected all sensations from her body which might remind her of the fact. She cut off awareness in her body, and in that sense was "out of touch." Such contradictory self-concepts can be seen in the woman who complains about how fat she is, yet refuses to look in a mirror or shop for clothes because she does not want to be confronted with seeing her body. As long as she does not "see" her body she does not have to accept the fat as there. We will develop this concept of "accepting the fat" later in the chapter.

Negative judgments about a woman's body are also derived from pervasive cultural concepts which deal with the "dirtiness" or "sinfulness" of the body. Women learn early that their bodies, especially their genitals, are dirty. Purity resides in the mind and soul. Furthermore, little girls learn that it is not nice to touch their bodies, to feel themselves. Their genitals, out of view for the most part, are rarely seen. A little girl generally has little opportunity to look at her vagina, her vulva, her clitoris, and so grows up with an unclear notion of what "down there" is all about. Because it is unacceptable to look at and touch the body, and because a girl has little opportunity to do so, it is no wonder that so many of us grow up "out of touch" with our bodies, no matter what our weight.

We live in a culture that not only teaches many of us that our bodies and the body functions are "dirty," but which often encourages us to distrust our body signals. Since the development of body image is dependent, in part, on our ability to perceive and identify internal body signals, it is not surprising that we have unclear body images. How much experience have we had in listening to the myriad signals which emanate from the body and which provide us with information as to our needs? Of course, in some areas, such awareness is allowed, even insisted upon — especially in heeding one's body's signals that it needs to defecate or urinate. Yet, there are thousands of other internal signals of which we are consciously unaware because we have not learned nor have we been encouraged to perceive and identify them. This being "out of touch" with our body signals leads to many disturbances in our eating behavior, as well, and we will explore this area in the chapter on "Eating Awareness."

The general distrust of the body leads us to attempt to regulate it through conscious will and to look to others, to authorities, to interpret what we feel or to even *tell* us what we feel. This attitude of distrust of the body contributes to our being "out of touch" with ourselves. Even deeper than distrust, one can often identify real fear of the body. We live in a culture which sees the mind and body as split, and which strives to have the conscious mind gain as much control as possible over the body. The conscious willful mind is viewed as the rightful master and is often perceived as our "real" selves. Anything not under the control of the conscious mind is suspect and an object of fear. Even the concept that we have an unconscious mind which influences how we think, feel, and act makes many of us uncomfortable, because it implies a lack of control—control being the conscious will of the mind. Yet, in reality, the conscious mind is not "all," is not even the master, nor is the mind separate from the body. Despite one's religious or philosophical orientation, one must accept at the very least that the mind and body are in a complex and intimate relationship with one another and are constantly interacting.

Your conscious mind is not the final master but only part of you. Most of your life processes are carried on at an unconscious level without any conscious attention. The "real" you does not reside in your mind. You are the totality of your mind and body.

Rather than disown your body, because it is frightening and not always amenable to conscious control, it is helpful to get to know your body, get "in touch" with it, make peace with it. Instead of fearing the body, you will begin to see that the various sensations that arise from the body are signals and messages about your needs or even your present emotional state.

Emotions, be they anger, joy or fear, all have physical components in the body. There are certain measurable changes in the body—in blood pressure, hormonal activity, muscular activity—which accompany the feeling of fear, for instance. This is known as the fight/flight response, in which the body reacts to perceived fear by gearing up for a fight or a flight away from danger. Anger can raise the blood pressure and tighten the muscles. We all know the pleasant body sensations of joy.

These bodily sensations which accompany emotions can often provide us with clues as to our emotional state. The tightening of jaw muscles or a clenched fist can clue us into anger of which we have been unaware. One patient with whom I worked came to realize that whenever she got a headache, it meant that she was upset with something her husband had done or said and she needed to talk to him. Once she decided to talk to him the headache would disappear.

Ivy Helstein, a teacher of assertiveness training, once told a group of women in her workshop that each time a person does not assert herself in a situation, each time she says "yes" when the true desire was to say "no," there is a physical reaction, a twinge in the body, often in the gut or the stomach. It is a barely perceptible sensation, but it is there, and it is my belief that often a woman will misinterpret this bodily sensation as a sign of hunger. How often might we be eating because we never learned to distinguish between or interpret just such normal bodily sensations? There are so many messages being sent from our muscles, our organs, our skin. How much more peaceful an existence we could have if we could learn to "read" these messages and learn to heed them, so that our conscious minds could work with these body sensations, not against them.

Since it is the purpose of this chapter to help you develop a sense of body awareness as it relates to your eating problem, I will not present any exercises which focus on general body awareness, but instead will refer you to the bibliography which contains several good books with body awareness exercises. The chapter on "Eating Awareness" will focus specifically on developing your ability to identify and listen to those bodily sensations which signal hunger and fullness.

For now, let us return to the issue of the distorted body image. By distorted body image I mean the distorted or disturbed picture a woman has about what she looks like or her size. It is reflected in the statements: "I can feel both fat and thin in a single day!" "Sometimes when I look in the mirror, I don't know who that person is staring back." "People tell me I'm fat, but I don't feel it." "People tell me I'm getting too thin, but I still feel fat."

The most dramatic example of distorted body image occurs in the anorectic who claims, despite her bony, emaciated appearance, that she is still overweight, but such disturbed thinking is present to a lesser degree in almost all compulsive eaters. Most women with bulimia are obsessed with thinness, and though unlike anorectics they are usually within "normal" weight ranges, many such women continue to perceive themselves as fat. No amount of encouragement or statements to the contrary from those around them will change their perceptions. Obese women will often view themselves as much heavier or even thinner than they actually are. It is clear that the intensity of dissatisfaction and misperception of one's body size is not merely a function of degree of overweight.

What leads to such distorted self-perceptions? Again, it is possible that the negative judgments which contribute to unclear body images underlie, as well, the distorted body images so many of us possess. If a woman comes to view her body in a negative light, she may begin to disassociate herself from it, and not only may she be unable to form a clear picture of her body in her mind, but the picture she does form is likely to be inaccurate and distorted. In addition, by focusing her displeasure on body parts which she finds unacceptable, the woman may be exaggerating the prominence of these parts in forming her self-image. Hence the statement: "When I walk onto a tennis court, I think everyone is looking at my fat thighs," made by a woman who most people would say is thin and attractive. In her mind, and in her body image, those "fat" thighs stick out as a most distinctive feature. How did this woman come to view herself this way? Perhaps at one time she did have heavy thighs and has never adjusted her body image to the weight loss; or perhaps someone once inadvertently referred to her thighs as heavy (in proportion to the rest of her body); or she may even have overheard someone talking about someone's fat thighs and mistakenly assumed that the person was speaking of her.

Women who have been overweight since childhood or adolescence generally have the most difficulty adjusting their perceptions of their size to their actual weight loss. When body concepts were being formed, the feedback received from others led them to include "fat" as part of their image. Once their body image is firmly established, weight loss alone is not enough to effect a change in the image. In my readings and in my practice, I have come across numerous examples of women who have lost huge amounts of weight, but still view themselves as fat. One such woman continued to look at large sizes in clothing stores, though she no longer needed them. In fact, she was quite slender. Yet she often "forgot" she had lost weight and would head straight for the large sizes in a store. Similarly, many women who have been heavy all their lives and then lose large amounts of weight have trouble identifying with the thin images they see in the mirror. They still feel and expect to see themselves as fat. If, in the chapter on "The Power of Fat," your fat/thin list included "me" under the fat heading, such a distorted body image is likely to result when you do lose weight.

Other women manifest their distorted body images in disassociating themselves from their fat, acting as if it is not there. Especially in an obese woman, the negative judgments about her body—both from others and from herself—can lead her to reject her fat and see herself as thin. This phenomenon was evidenced in a patient of mine who repeatedly saw the scales as registering one hundred pounds lower than she actually weighed. Although on some level she knew she was really obese, on another level she rejected the fat as "not there." She often was shocked upon glimpsing her passing reflection in a store window. What she saw was a fat woman. Inside she felt thin.

Rejection of one's fat is present in most women with eating problems, though most of us reject our fat not in being unaware of its existence, but in not accepting it, wanting to disassociate ourselves from it. That rejection underlies our reluctance to look at ourselves in the mirror or to shop for clothes in a larger size. For one woman, to shop for clothes meant "the final acceptance, the realization, the unmistakable proof that I've gained weight." There is a reluctance, even a fear in accepting one's fat. What is this reluctance about? In part, it may stem from the fact that gaining weight and being fat, for most of us, is an unpleasant and painful experience, and from a natural desire to avoid thinking about or dealing with something which makes us unhappy. Yet it is my experience that this reluctance to accept one's fat, to "own" it, has deeper roots. When asked, "What are you afraid would happen if you just accepted the fat you have on your body as yours without judging yourself harshly?" my patients have given interesting responses. Some are afraid that if they accept their fat, own up to its existence, they will have to do something about it. "I'll have to take responsibility for it." "I will have to go on a diet or begin an exercise program, or something I don't want to do, if I begin to 'own' my fat, to acknowledge its existence. I'd rather not think about it, pretend it isn't there." Remember that when we refer to "accepting" or "owning" our fat, we do not mean to imply that women are unaware that they have the fat on their bodies. In fact, in some ways many women are overaware and self-conscious about the fat on their bodies; yet at the same time they also reject the fat, refuse to accept it as their own. This is a difficult concept, but the meaning will become clearer as you begin to analyze your perceptions in the exercise which follows.

For some women the idea of "owning" one's fat, of accepting its existence on the body without making negative judgments, evokes another kind of fear. This fear is exemplified in the following common statement: "If I just accept the fat on my body, and I don't hate myself for being fat, why will I ever lose weight? If I don't reject it, what will motivate me to lose it?" Many assume you have to hate the fat in order to get rid of it, as though hatred of fat and of yourself for gaining it is the only motivation you have to give it up. Think again. Think of what you learned in the last chapter on "The Reality of Thin." You have realistic reasons to want to give up the weight—health reasons or desires to move and breathe more easily, the prospect of a greater variety of clothes to chose from, and so on. These reasons, not self-hate, will be your real motivations for giving up the weight. In fact, self-hate is unlikely to bring about weight loss, because the response of most compulsive eaters to such negative emotions is to eat. How often have you responded to a weight gain with self-hate and then with even more eating? Acceptance of the weight without judgment can lead to a clearer examination of what you have been doing with food and why you might have needed to put on more weight (what function the fat is serving). Such an examination of your actions in gaining weight is more likely to lead to eventual loss of the fat.

There is yet another reason why accepting and "owning" one's fat is so important, and though I heard Susie Orbach and Carol

Munter repeat it often when I was in their group, it took me many months to really understand it. That reason is that "You cannot lose something you don't own." If the fat on your body is not "there" in your mind, or if it feels like something apart from you, temporarily placed on your body, you cannot lose it. You need to "own" it, to accept its existence as part of you, and to own its functions and uses in order to be able to give it up. If it is not yours, it is not yours to give up. The work of the second chapter helped you "own" the functions fat has been serving in your life. The exercises in this chapter will help you "own" your fat in the sense of feeling it as a part (but only a part) of you.

It is ironic that while on one level women with compulsive eating problems identify themselves through their fat and are overly conscious of others' reactions to their fat, on another level, they see their fat as not a part of them. Women with fat on their bodies (no matter how much fat they actually possess) tend to see the fat as covering the "real" me. The following examples illustrate my point:

> Recently a local newspaper carried an ad for a diet center program which pictured a thin woman stepping out from within a fat body. It looked like she had just zipped the fat body down and walked out—as though the fat was not the real her. There is a common expression that inside every fat person lives a thin one dying to get out.
>
> A woman in one of my groups got in touch with her fear that if she lost weight "people could get too close to me. There'd be no fat between me and them. Now I have the fat to keep them at a distance. They can never get to the 'real me.' "

The reality is that there is no "real" you "inside." You are the totality of all that is contained within your skin. Your fat is part of you. No one can get any closer to you than the limits of your body—whether those limits are wide and include much fat within them or the limits become narrower as you give up some of the fat. This knowledge is crucial to being able to give up your fat permanently. If you view the fat as protective covering, to give it up would leave you feeling vulnerable and frightened. The work of this chapter focuses to a large extent on extending your concept of yourself, the "real you," to the limits of your body—including your fat within.

When we speak of extending your self-concept to the limits of your body, we are moving into the area of your body image which concerns a felt sense of your boundary or borders. Usually we do not give much thought to the concept of our boundaries, yet we have all developed such a concept. In his book, *Body Consciousness*, Seymour Fisher writes, "If you ask the average person about his body boundary, you will only get a puzzled look. While he knows that all structures have walls and defining limits, he has probably never applied this idea to his own body. If pressed, he will admit, 'of course, there are boundaries to my body. My body is enclosed by skin and that skin marks the edge of me.' But he is rarely aware that he has learned basic attitudes about 'the edge of me' and whether it is substantial and defensible . . . the average person does not become aware of his sense of possessing a psychologically defined body boundary and its potent functions until something happens to him that seriously disturbs these functions."[2] He cites examples of people who experience brain damage and lose the ability to distinguish between what is happening inside them from events on the outside. Schizophrenics and people under the influence of certain hallucinogenic drugs often experience a similar breaking down of the boundaries.

Women, especially those with compulsive eating problems, often have an unclear sense of defined borders which can be defended. Our training has taught us to be empathetic, to care for and merge with others, to extend our psychological boundaries out to include our children, husbands, friends. When we give so much of ourselves to others, we may be unclear about where we begin and where we end. When we are unclear about our psychological boundaries and also see fat as something apart from and surrounding our bodies, then we cannot give up the fat. Ironically, the fat both provides a thick boundary or border of protection and, at the same time, makes our boundaries seem more ambiguous, more unclear. We are lost in a sea of fat. Some women have expressed their fear of being thin, because a thin body has such clearly defined lines—unlike the flowing, ambiguous lines of a fat body.

In an article, "Never Too Thin To Feel Fat," Judith Thurman examined her feelings about fat and thin: "Being fat has also nourished in me a sense of grandiosity about isolation. The fatness, like a long deep bitter winter has been comfortable to dream through. And strangely, the fatter I am the more safe and invisible I feel; the flesh blurs me—just as being thin defines my edges in relation to the world. Thin, I stand outlined and exposed. You can see me and touch me, which I want, but which is also frightening."[3]

Let us now turn to an exercise which will help elucidate the concept of boundaries as well as that of "owning" the fat. This is the "mirror exercise"—one which is as important as it is difficult to do. Briefly, it will consist merely of looking at yourself in a mirror, daily, without judgments about the way you look. Most women find this a difficult task at first, but eventually it becomes interesting, even adventurous.

Mirror Exercises

This exercise requires you to set aside some time, each day, to look at yourself, preferably without clothes, in a full length, accurate mirror. You will be asked throughout the exercise to observe and examine yourself without critical evaluations or judgments. Remember, I am asking you to learn to accept your fat—not love it, but accept it. Remember too that you have not put this fat on your body to be self-destructive or to punish. The fat is not a sin. You have this fat on your body because it has been doing something for you (it serves a function), and because you have used food to meet emotional needs. Accepting the fat without critical judgment is the first step toward giving it up. When you do the exercise each day, do one or more of the following steps:

1. Look at yourself in the mirror. Try to get a sense of where you end and the world begins. Look at your arms. See the outline of those arms as defining where you end and the rest of the world

begins. Look at your torso, your hips, your legs. See the outlines of this body.
2. Now, look at each part of your body in relation to the other parts. See how the arms are attached to the shoulders, the shoulders to the torso, and so on. See the proportions of your body. What is the size of your hips in proportion to your chest or your shoulders? Get a sense of the structure of your body.
3. Now, feel your body. Touch your face, your arms, shoulders, chest, hips, back. Feel the skin. Trace the outlines of your body as you look. You might reaffirm to yourself, "This is me. This is all of me."
4. Look at yourself from all angles. Move around and see what you look like from the side, the back. Sit down on the floor and look at your vagina, your clitoris. (Some women use more than one mirror at various angles to view their bodies from different perspectives.)
5. Turn on some music you especially like and move around to the music. Watch your body as you move. (One woman used candles and special lighting to create a special atmosphere to move in. She also took up belly dancing and practiced daily in front of the mirror.)

Discussion of Mirror Exercises

Although the purpose of these exercises may not be immediately apparent, the benefits are indeed many. First of all, the exercises will help you become more aware of your size and shape and your boundaries. As you trace the outlines of your body and differentiate your body from the background, your sense of having firm borders will slowly increase. Touching is a good way to get a felt sense of the boundaries of your body.

Especially if they are done in a relaxed, nonjudgmental atmosphere, these exercises will enable you to begin accepting your fat as a part of you — to "own" your fat, rather than seeing it as a covering over the "real" you. In *Fat is a Feminist Issue*, Susie Orbach presents a diagram of three figures which illustrates the progressive steps of "growing into" one's body, so that when women lose weight they "will not feel that they are losing a protective covering, they grow into their bodies and then they will feel that they have their whole bodies which they can then afford to compress."[4]

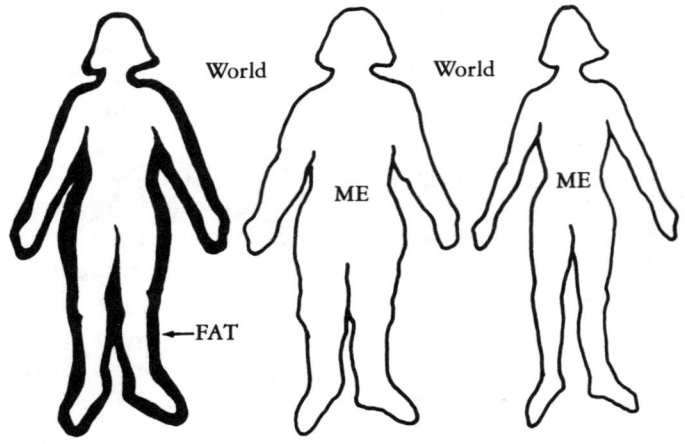

Unless you can integrate your fat into your body image, to lose it is to lose a barrier between yourself and the world. Once you have accepted your fat as within you and you have a clear sense of your boundaries you can lose the excess fat within your cells. You are not giving up anything. You are compacting, shrinking those expanded cells.

There is yet another important function these mirror exercises perform, and that is that they help you prepare for and adjust to weight loss, especially for those who have a number of pounds to lose. As we have seen, people who lose a lot of weight often have difficulty readjusting their body concepts. Most overweight women tend to avoid looking at themselves in the mirror, but after having lost weight, they begin looking. There is often a twinge of discomfort at the sight of their new thin body. "Who is this person? It doesn't feel like me," some women have exclaimed. There is a sense that one is living temporarily in a borrowed body that is unfamiliar, and it is not surprising that at some level there is a desire to escape this strange body and return to one which is comfortable and familiar and fat. This is where the mirror work can pay off. If you have lost fifty pounds over the past year, but have been monitoring and adjusting to the changes in your body daily, the thin body will not look dramatically different to you. An analogy would be the situation in which one sees a child for the first time in a year. The child may have grown so much in that year that she looks drastically different. Yet the parents, who saw her daily, had time to adjust to the gradual changes in her size, and are not as struck by the difference. Such is the case when you are losing weight and observing the changes daily. By the time you have lost your fifty pounds, you have slowly made adjustments to the changes in your body. You will not look in the mirror one day and suddenly be confronted with a body you do not know.

The next fantasy will also help you extend your body concept to include your fat. It is a fantasy which must be done several times before its benefits become apparent.

Expansion of Self Fantasy

Imagine that you are alone in your house. Nobody is around and you will have this time to yourself . . . undisturbed. . . . Now imagine yourself standing in front of your mirror without any clothes. . . . Look carefully at your body, nonjudgmentally. See if you can examine it as though it were a piece of sculpture in a museum. . . . Notice how all the parts fit together—how the head is attached to the neck, neck to shoulders, and so on. (Pause thirty seconds.) . . . Now breathe all the air out of your lungs. Keeping the image of yourself in your mind, slowly inhale, letting your stomach expand as you do so. . . . Hold your breath a second, then let it out slowly through your mouth. . . . Now, inhale again, expanding your stomach, this time becoming aware of the air coming into your body and reaching all parts of your body. See the image of the air filling you out to your extremities. . . . Exhale. Try this again, feeling the air flow into your fingertips, your toes, your head. (Pause twenty seconds.) . . . Very often our view of ourselves is that there is a "real me" somewhere inside. The fat is a covering, a protection, an annoyance, but somehow, something we reject and do not see as a part of ourselves. It is very hard to lose the fat permanently when you view yourself this way. So . . . looking at yourself again in the mirror, try to expand your image of yourself to include all of your body. As the air travels out to your extremities, let your concept of yourself, your essence, the real you, expand and fill out your whole body. Look at yourself again. . . . Walk around the room. Can you feel your body as more whole, more connected? Stay with this feeling for a while, checking out your image in the mirror or walking around. . . . And when you feel ready open your eyes and come back to your existence in the room.

Discussion of Expansion of Self

This fantasy is primarily an experiential one, and does not require analysis. However, I would like to repeat that its benefits in helping you to "own" your fat are often not apparent until the fantasy is done several times. One variation of the fantasy is to follow it up until the part where you are asked to look at yourself a second time, and then to open your eyes and actually look at yourself in a mirror, and walk around, feeling the sense of connectedness and wholeness described in the fantasy. The more you can integrate your fat into your sense of "self" the less distorted and unclear your body image will be.

The next exercise was designed to be done in a group setting, in which each woman draws a picture of what she thinks she looks like. No names are written on the drawings, but instead they are passed among the group members, who try to guess whose drawing they are looking at. Sometimes the drawings are accurate and are easy to identify. Other times, a drawing can reflect such an inaccurate or distorted view of the woman that no one can figure out to whom it belongs. Since most of you using this book will be working alone, two suggestions as to how to do this exercise are offered. First, you may do your drawing and then ask a trusted friend or family member or several others to evaluate your representation of yourself. It would be helpful to ask several people to make sure that you are getting objective feedback. For his or her own reasons, one person might have misperceptions or a distorted view of how you look. Several observers would cancel out such distortions. Alternatively, you may choose to work on your own, without outside input. In that case, it is especially important to have an accurate full-length mirror on hand.

Drawing of Self

1. Make a drawing of yourself, naked, including all the parts of your body you wish. It is not important that your drawing be aesthetically pleasing. The aim of this exercise is to draw your size and shape as accurately as possible.
2. When you have completed your drawing, you have the following options. You may choose one or both of them:
    a. Put the drawing away for a day or two. This will allow you to put some distance between yourself and the drawing in order to look at it more objectively. When you feel ready, take it out and look at it as a representation of what you think you look like. Keep the following questions in mind. While considering the questions it will be necessary to compare your reflection in a full length mirror—its size, shape, proportions—to the image depicted in the drawing.
       1) Is this picture an accurate representation of what I look like?
       2) Have I drawn any particular body parts larger than they really are or larger in proportion to the rest of my body than they really are?
       3) Are there any body parts conspicuous by their absence? This can tell you something about how you feel about your body, and about parts you might be trying to "disown." If there were any body parts left out, ask yourself "why?"
    b. Show the drawing to one or several other people. Ask them if they view it as an accurate representation of your body. You might have them consider the above questions in forming their opinions.

Discussion of Drawing of Self

It is not surprising, given the unclear and distorted body images women often possess, that many women's drawings reflect inaccurate perceptions such as viewing the body as much fatter or thinner than it is, or exaggerating the prominence of one particular body part in relation to the others.

Let us look at some examples of how women in my groups have represented themselves. The following drawings are my own reproductions of their work. They are sufficiently accurate, however, for the purposes of this book.

Drawing #1 Toby

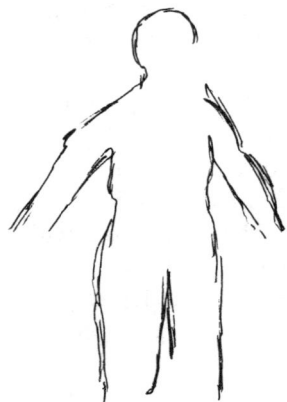

The most striking characteristic of Toby's drawing is the indistinctness of its lines. There are no feet, no hands, no features, and the lines of the body are so ambiguous that one has no sense of a distinct body clearly separate from its surroundings. She seems almost to melt into the background. My first impression of this representation was that Toby was a woman with no clear sense of personal boundaries. Further exploration revealed Toby's lack of identity, her feeling that she was "nothing." Her orientation to the world was to try to please everyone. She lived through her children and her husband, feeling she derived identity from them. She gave of herself to everyone, rarely thinking of herself. You could say that she had a poor sense of psychological boundaries, extending her concept of self to include all those around her. Her unclear physical sense of boundaries was a reflection of her psychological state. She viewed her fat as providing her with substance and protection. It kept her from melting into the background. Based on insights gained from analyzing her picture, Toby felt she needed to develop an identity of her own apart from her family, and to establish a sense of distinct physical boundaries. In order to firm up her sense of having distinct physical boundaries which delineated her separateness from the rest of the world, Toby increased her mirror work, especially focusing on touching her body. She also took up yoga.

Drawing #2 Marsha

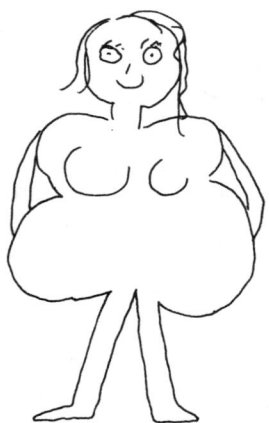

Marsha's drawing is typical of women who see their fat as merely covering their true selves. The head, legs and arms are of normal size and the fat appears to be stuck on a thin body. It is clear from this drawing that Marsha does not "own" her fat, but sees it as a covering, ballooning out over her "real" skinny body. It is also not a far-fetched inference that Marsha sees her fat as protecting her in some way.

Drawing #3 Marjorie

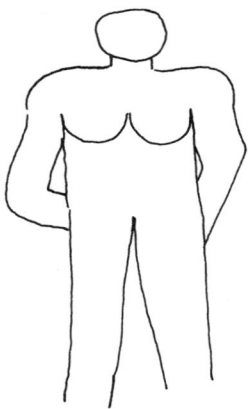

The masculine quality of Marjorie's drawing was surprising. While obese, Marjorie had a body that looked feminine and rounded. Other words that entered my mind upon seeing *this* body were "powerful," "Frankenstein's Monster," "solid," "steel." Evidently Marjorie saw herself this way, and perhaps she *needed* to see herself as huge and powerful. She had had an unusually difficult life and was currently involved in a situation which required all her strength. Perhaps she thought she needed the fat to make her large and powerful. A thin, feminine body might have seemed inadequate to handle the constant burdens and crises of her life. Yet the reality was that Marjorie's remarkable strength (and she *was* strong) was not derived from her body at all, but from a deep inner emotional strength. It was Marjorie's task to come to "own" that inner strength rather than attribute it to her fat.

Checking out your own drawing for inaccurate perception of your proportions can be enlightening. One of the women in my groups, Sara, had always believed herself to be broad-shouldered. A relative had told her once when Sara was a child that she had inherited the family tendency toward broad shoulders, and so Sara had incorporated this relative's perception of her body into her body image. When she drew herself for this exercise, she did indeed draw herself as she perceived herself to be—with large shoulders "like a football player"—but *Sara did not have broad shoulders*. The only way she could be convinced of this fact was by looking at herself objectively and noncritically in the mirror, checking out the width of her shoulders as compared to the width of her waist and hips. She was amazed to discover that her body was evenly proportioned, and was surprised that she had carried this misperception around within her for so many years. The inaccurate body image had been reflected in the way she drew herself.

Look back at your own drawings. Perhaps you can now begin to get a sense of what your drawing is telling you about the way you view your body and your fat.

It would be a good idea to repeat this exercise several months from now. As you develop your body concept more fully, the changes will be reflected in your new drawings.

The next exercise requires you to get a large piece of paper—large enough to trace your body. If you cannot find such paper, improvise by piecing together a few sheets. You will also need someone to do the tracing.

Outline of Self

Lie down on the paper you have prepared, preferably without any clothing. If you must wear something, try to make it the thinnest, most body-hugging piece of clothing you own. Position yourself on the paper so that your legs are slightly apart and your arms are out away from your body. Now have someone take a pencil or crayon and trace the outlines of your body.

Discussion of Outline of Self

The purpose of this exercise is to help you gain a more accurate picture of the outlines and contours of your body. Sometimes even the mirror exercises or the drawing of yourself are not sufficient to correct a distorted body concept. Seeing the bare outlines of your body can give you a clearer sense of your size, how much space you take up, your shape, and the proportions of your body. Perhaps, as Sara the "broad-shouldered" woman discovered, you have been exaggerating the prominence of certain body features and thus perceiving yourself as looking very different from the way you actually look to the world.

Aluminum Foil Exercise

There is one last exercise you might try. It was devised by a patient of mine and provides an ingenious method of viewing how your body looks to the outside world. Wrap aluminum foil around your body, from the neck down to the upper legs. You must put several layers of aluminum foil around you, so that you will be able to create a shape solid enough to stand up when you are no longer inside it. It might be a good idea to enlist the help of another. Once you have wrapped yourself firmly in the foil, cut an opening down the back, so you can slip out of it. Once you are out, try to piece the back together. You will now have an empty shell. Fill the foil up with crumpled newspapers to help hold the shape. Now you have created a form which roughly matches your own in size and shape. The patient who developed the idea for this exercise used the form in various ways to give herself a clear picture of how her body looked to others. She placed it in various chairs in her home and looked at it from different angles. She even brought the form to one of our sessions and placed it on the couch to see how much space she took up when she sat there. This exercise, unlike the others, gives you a three-dimensional view of yourself and therefore a better sense of your size.

The concept of how much space one takes up is an important one, and these exercises are not mere games. As we saw from the analysis of Marjorie's drawing of herself, sometimes a woman may need to perceive herself (or actually *be*) large in order to withstand hardships in her life. Or she may, like Toby, perceive herself as lacking identity and importance. A large body gives her substance, even presence. Are you making a statement to yourself, to the world, with a large body? Do you need to perceive yourself as large? How would you feel in a smaller, narrower body?

Remember, the purpose of all these exercises in this chapter is to increase your accurate awareness of your body size and shape. I am not asking you to love your body, but to accept it for what it is. It is important to feel comfortable with yourself, at any weight.

Ironically, accepting one's weight realistically and noncritically is a first step toward being able to give it up.

The rest of this chapter will focus on two aspects of bodywork which can help you in the process of learning more about your body—the uses of clothing, and of exercise.

We touched on the subject of clothes in our earlier discussion of things you are putting off until you get thin. Though it is not necessary to focus attention on clothing in order to give up one's fat, there is much to gain from an examination of the symbolic meanings and uses of clothes.

In one sense the clothes one chooses to wear can be seen as presenting messages about the wearer. Clothes can be viewed as part of a self-portrait, a definition of self. The woman who chooses to wear designer jeans is telling the world something about herself, very different from what another woman is saying by wearing overalls. Think for a moment. What messages are you sending to the world through your wardrobe?

"I wear what I can find in my large size," says one woman. "I wear what I can afford," says another. Yet, perhaps there is more to your choice of clothes than you realize. For instance, one obese woman may choose clothes in bright, happy colors or of interesting prints, while another, the same weight, may choose only grays, beiges, and browns. The way in which the clothes are worn can say something about you as well. The first woman may wear exotic or unusual jewelry to complement her bright yellow shirt. The second woman may wear her wrinkled beige top with a button missing. The first woman may feel good about herself and feel deserving of looking good—no matter what her weight. The second woman may be saying to the world, "I don't think much of myself" or, "I don't feel deserving of looking good, because I'm fat" or, "Don't notice me." Whatever the message, it is helpful to discover what you have been saying to the world with your clothes, why you might want to be giving this message, and explore whether you do, in fact, want to be sending that message.

Just as clothes define you to the rest of the world, they also have messages for *you*. You could be using clothing to control your behavior. In the chapter on fat we learned that a woman could be using her fat to control her sexual desires, so that she would be sure she would not "fool around." The choice of clothing can have a similar function. You may choose clothing that hides your shape, so that you will not be seen as sexual. This use of clothing can be very positive, since it can perform the same function as the fat, allowing you to be thin, but giving you a sense of control over yourself. Though your fantasy of yourself as thin may include beautiful sexy clothing, perhaps for some of you a loose, baggy wardrobe may be necessary.

Clothing can also provide you with the opportunity to examine whom you would *like* to be. Wearing different kinds of clothes enables you to check out what it would feel like to be a certain way — experiencing what it would be like to perceive oneself or be perceived differently. Perhaps my experience will best illustrate this process. When I was "fat," I wore only skirts, because I thought I looked too heavy in pants. The outfits I chose were nondescript, standard skirts and blouses. In my mind I had always pictured myself thin, wearing exotic jewelry and peasant blouses with long skirts or slacks. I would not allow myself to wear such clothes unless I got thin; yet there was nothing keeping me from wearing such clothes. Finally, I decided to express this more exotic part of my personality by wearing one of the outfits I had always dreamed of wearing when I got thin. I decided not to wait until I had lost weight and I quickly made the outfit from a colorful print material. It consisted of a long flared skirt, with a peasant blouse, long necklaces, sandals, and on my head, a scarf made of the same material as the skirt. I looked like a gypsy, but that was exactly the image I wanted to create — as though by wearing these clothes I was saying to the world, "This is a part of me you don't often see, but this exotic, different part is there nonetheless." I wanted to stand out. I tested out the clothing slowly, first wearing it to my group, getting feedback, and then wearing the outfit to work. I began to feel comfortable with the image I was projecting, and was especially pleased that I had learned to express something about myself through clothes rather than through fat or eating. I still occasionally wear similar outfits, though I now possess a wardrobe which is expressive of many different parts of my personality.

It would be a good idea to explore how you can express yourself through clothing, irrespective of whether you are losing weight or not. You might, like me, discover that you feel comfortable in new kinds of clothing, with different messages, or you may find that the image you had always hoped to create when you got thin, just is not for you. One of my patients, Linda, had always pictured herself wearing short shorts and a tiny tank top when she got thin. Though she was not able to find such clothing in her size, I urged her to experiment with wearing revealing or sexy clothing at her present weight. She was able to find a very attractive, low-cut blouse which fit her well, but she felt very uncomfortable wearing it to group. At first, she thought the discomfort was merely self-consciousness about her fat, but when I asked her to envision herself thin and wearing the same blouse, she became aware that she would feel uneasy exposing her body. She did not want people to be looking down her blouse, or staring at her large breasts. What Linda discovered was that even if she were thin, she would not feel comfortable wearing revealing, tight-fitting clothing. This realization unburdened her and decreased her fear about getting thin, because she had believed that when she became thin she would have to or want to wear such clothing.

For some women, especially those with boundary problems, tight-fitting clothing can be perceived not as revealing but as helping to define the lines, boundaries, and limits of one's body. Large, flowing clothes can make one appear less defined and can be used in situations in which the desire is to appear ambiguous or to blend in.

For one woman with whom I worked, Natalie, clothing provided the same protective function her fat had served in the past. For months she wore a heavy down vest. When she felt vulnerable and in need of protection she would keep it on. When she felt safe and comfortable, she would take it off. Natalie referred to her vest as "my portable fat."

Again, consider how you have been using clothing to send messages to yourself and the world. How could you make changes which would make those messages more clear and effective? Or do you want to explore what it would be like to send different messages? Remember you can see what it is like to project sexiness or assertiveness or sophistication through your choice of clothing, and if you do not feel comfortable with the message you can always change your clothes.

Some of my patients have protested at my suggestion that they experiment with clothes, because of lack of funds or because of the limited selection of clothes in their sizes. It is surely not my intent that you invest large sums of money in new clothing, and I realize that for those of you who are obese your choice of clothes may be severely limited (though many stores are beginning to carry attractive and interesting clothes in extra-large sizes as women begin to demand change). What I propose is that you give some thought to projecting a self-identity through the clothing you wear—creating a distinctive look. This may mean wearing certain kinds of jewelry, for instance. I had always envisioned myself wearing long earrings when I got "thin." Since I never got thin enough, I never bought the earrings. Then one day, while in my group, I decided to get my ears pierced. In the years since then I have come to be known for the unusual earrings I've collected from all over the world. The earrings and other jewelry I choose distinguish me, make a statement about me in a way I had always used my fat to do. You may begin to create your own identity in small ways: buying a blouse in a style or color different from what you usually buy, or changing your hairstyle. Those of you who sew can make yourselves the kinds of clothes you wish to wear, so that even if local stores do not carry your size, you can experiment with different styles. If you have always wanted to wear a long skirt, but the stores do not have them in large sizes, make one.

Let us turn now to the issue of exercise and how it can help you establish a better sense of body image; but first I must make it clear that it is not necessary that you exercise in order to lose weight. Exercise has many benefits, both in terms of weight loss and in improving distorted or unclear body concepts, but is it fruitless to tell a person she *should* exercise. The desire to exercise has to come from some inner need to move the body and to master certain movements. No amount of exhortation will move the unwilling. No discussions of the benefits will motivate someone who does not like to or want to participate in physical activity to get out and run. However, taking up some form of exercise can have so many benefits for your emotional and physical well-being, I thought it important to include a discussion of exercise in this chapter on Bodywork.

In my own inner journey, exercise was essential to my work in learning about myself and learning to feel comfortable with my body. I even found a joy in moving my body. Other women with whom I have worked have expressed similar sentiments.

For a woman with an inadequate concept of her boundaries, various forms of physical activity can strengthen her sense of body boundaries. In *Body Consciousness*, Seymour Fisher writes that "we have found in our laboratory that we can exercise some control over the boundary by instructing people to focus their attention on specific body areas. For example, we can augment the boundary by getting them to increase their awareness of skin and muscles. This can be done by deliberate control of attention or by engaging in exercises that activate skin and muscle . . . there are already several studies that show that schizophrenic patients can be helped for brief periods to firm up their borders by being given tasks that increase their skin and muscle awareness."[5]

Yoga is one form of exercise in which the focus of attention is on the area of the body being stretched during a pose. The benefits in firming up one's sense of boundaries through the practice of yoga can be enormous though any movement which helps increase your awareness of your skin and muscles will perform the same function.

In the chapter on Eating Awareness, we will work on developing the ability to listen to and trust one's own internal body signals. There is a natural body wisdom which can be relied on to tell you what your body needs at any given time. Before you begin to focus on the inner sensations which signal hunger or fullness, it is important to learn to identify and trust the body signals in general. Exercise can help you tap into this inner body wisdom. Active participation in a sport or exercise program gives you a sense of your body you have probably never had before. For example, a runner learns quickly when it is time to push her body to its limits and when it is time to pull back and rest. As she begins to trust her body to tell her what it needs, she may begin to trust that her body can give messages as to its food needs as well. "Maybe I can trust my body to tell me what, when and how much food it needs to eat, just as it tells me what it needs when I'm running," said one of my patients who had taken up running while she was in her group.

Most women have had little experience with sports as little girls, and have not learned some of the lessons which their male counterparts learned as a matter of course—comfort and trust in the body's ability to signal its needs, for example. Little boys learn through physical activity when to push themselves and when their bodies are signaling for rest. As we encourage our daughters to be active in sports, they too should grow up with a sense of trust in their bodies.

There is also a sense of mastery that comes from engaging in a sport or exercise program—a feeling that you can move your body in any way you want, that you have the flexibility and strength to do with your body as you will. From my various exercises, I have gained a sense of mastery of my muscles, a body awareness, a feeling of wholeness that is not easily described.

Another possible benefit to be gained from engaging in physical exercise is weight loss. We all know that exercising can burn up calories and lead to weight loss, but the benefits to which I refer have to do with weight loss in individuals who find it difficult to lose. For many reasons, some people cannot get thin, or as thin as they would like to be. One of these reasons is relevant to our discussion here, but to understand the benefits of exercising for such people, let me first explain the concept of "set points." There is a theory that the body has a control system which regulates how much fat it will store. When the fat reserves in the body become too high, this system, like a thermostat, clicks on and attempts to lower the fat stores by reducing the appetite. Conversely, when the fat reserves get too low, the system increases the appetite in order to increase food intake and return to the set point weight. Your set point weight is probably the weight at which you spend most of your time. Though you may gain a few pounds or lose a few, you tend to move back toward your set point in time. There is increasing evidence to support this theory, though it is not clear how the theory accounts for individuals who keep getting heavier each year. Nonetheless, the set point theory can explain, in part, why many women are unable to lose those "last ten pounds" permanently.

An article in *Science 1982* had some interesting comments about the set point theory and how a person's set point can be lowered. Certain drugs such as amphetamines act on the brain, lowering the set point, but their effects are only temporary, and when the drugs are discontinued, the set point returns to normal. However, the one safe method that has been shown to lower the set point is physical conditioning, especially in those who are obese. Interestingly, inactivity tends to make normal weight individuals get heavier. No one knows why exercise lowers the set point, but the fact is that it does.[6]

It is my view that the human body was meant to move and that it functions best when it gets enough physical activity. The benefits of physical activity are emotional as well. There is increasing evidence, for example, that running (or any other aerobic activity) performed for a period of time has an effect on the brain chemistry, inducing the brain to produce certain hormones which elevate the mood. These studies have relevance for depressed individuals and indeed there are many psychotherapists who have their depressed patients on running programs in addition to traditional psychotherapy.

In *Getting Strong*, Kathryn Lance describes her experience with exercise and sports and their effects on her life. She talks about her involvement in physical exercise as setting off a domino effect: "In my own case, the first domino stood until I was thirty years old. At that time I was helpless, or believed myself to be, in nearly all areas of my life. I was a sedentary, overweight slave to cigarettes, fearful and nervous, dependent on those around me, and barely on speaking terms with my body. Then I began a running program, and the first domino fell. As I continued to run I discovered that even I, possibly the most unathletic person who ever lived, had a body capable of physical improvement and enjoyment. The self-confidence this discovery gave me enabled me to branch out physically, to take up a sport for the first time in my life and become good at it, to want to become strong, to further improve and integrate my body into my life. After the first flush of this new physical self-confidence, the dominos began rapidly falling in areas other than the physical: confidence in my body gave me mental and emotional confidence, and I began to venture into new avenues in my career."[7]

I hope this chapter will have given you a start, a beginning in working on your body concept and firming your sense of owning your body. In the next part of your journey you will be taking your new body awareness and focusing it on the specific area of eating—learning when you are hungry, when you are full, and what foods your body needs at any particular time. The work of this chapter should have prepared you to go on to this next area of eating awareness.

five

Eating Awareness

The newborn baby cries from hunger, and she is fed. When she has had enough, she stops eating, and all is well. Each newborn baby is a marvel of eating awareness. Each child knows, from the moment of birth, when she needs to eat and how much is required to ensure her growth. Later on, at times of rapid growth, she may seek extra food; yet when sick, nothing may appeal save water or juice. She knows when she has had enough and desires not a drop more.

The human body possesses an extraordinary self-regulatory mechanism—a system that is delicately balanced. This mechanism lets one know what, when, and how much food is needed to maintain optimum weight and health. It signals hunger and sends messages indicating degrees of fullness. Yet most adult compulsive eaters have been out of touch with these inner signals for so long that the delicate balance has been disrupted. They no longer heed nor even perceive the myriad messages their bodies send out about their inner needs. Furthermore, because the balance has been upset, the messages sent are often garbled or unclear.

How did this unfortunate state of affairs come about? How can the compulsive eater learn to interpret and respond to her inner body signals once again? How can the balance be restored? These questions form the basis of this chapter.

First, let us return to our newborn baby and explore what happens to her. We will call her Jenny. At the advice of her pediatrician. Jenny's mother puts her on a four-hour feeding schedule. Though her body may scream out for food, Jenny must wait until it is "time" to eat. At times, she is fed when she feels no hunger at all. Sometimes she is cajoled into drinking "just a little more" even though her body is clearly signaling "full." These early experiences are likely to confuse her.

As she grows, food begins to take on a special significance. Perhaps she is told that if she eats everything on her plate, she will get a treat, or a sweet may be offered to help ease the pain of a nasty fall. She may even be made to finish her plate, because of the starving children in _____. (Fill in the blank. Yes, that line is still being used.) The results of this early training are even more confusion and a slow process of learning to disregard natural feelings about food. She herself begins to use food to meet emotional needs.

At the same time, Jenny will likely be introduced to the pleasures of sugar in the form of candy, ice cream, and cookies. The huge amounts of refined sugar found in these and other common foods tend to further upset the delicate balance of the self-regulatory mechanism—particularly in certain individuals. The palate accustoms itself to extremely sweet foods, and loses its ability to discriminate the tastes of more natural, less sweet foods. (I am not implying here that one should never eat refined sugar, but merely that large amounts of sugar can upset the body's ability to discriminate and choose its foods.)

As Jenny enters the social world of twentieth century America, she learns to eat at specified hours, no matter what her body tells her, and she only eats certain foods at the appropriate time—chicken for breakfast? cereal for dinner? Never! Everything she has encountered so far has led Jenny to distrust and even disregard the natural inner signals her body sends as to its needs for food. However, if Jenny develops a weight problem, the confusion she has experienced so far is minimal compared to what is in store. First, she is *told* to disregard her body's messages. She is allowed to eat only specified foods at specified times. If pangs of hunger strike before mealtime she is supposed to exert all her will and suppress them. She is told not to trust her inner sensations, but to leave her eating decisions to another—the doctor or book or group which has put her on the diet. After years of such dieting, Jenny is totally out of touch and certainly distrustful of her body—and no wonder!

Your own situation is likely to be similar to Jenny's. It is likely that after years of dieting and gaining, it is hard to believe that you can trust your body to tell you what or how much food it needs. Yet, not only does your body "know" what it requires, it "knows" how to lose weight without dieting. By careful attention to one's inner signals, body weight can be normalized.

Let me state at the outset that I do not advocate dieting.[1] First of all, diets do not work—at least not in the long run. Whatever weight is lost on the diet is usually quickly regained, and each unsuccessful diet reinforces a sense of failure and weakness of character. It is discouraging to constantly view oneself as weak-willed. Yet diet failures are not the result of a weak will. Often, as we have seen, a woman has certain fears about what she will be like when she becomes thin. These fears often produce an eating binge. In some cases, a diet cannot be adhered to because food means too much to the dieter to be given up—food is used to meet many emotional needs which cannot be satisfied in any other way. As the eminent psychiatrist Hilde Bruch has written, the obese (and in *my* experience all compulsive eaters, no matter what their weight) "have in common the inability to identify hunger correctly or to distinguish it from other states of bodily need or emotional arousal. It became gradually clear that the old charge against obese people of having no will power describes their not being discriminately aware of bodily sensations: they cannot exercise control over a function or need which is not even recognized."[2]

Dieting is a form of self-deprivation, and the end result of an attempt at dieting is very often an enormous binge. The dieter deprives herself of the foods she loves—the very foods she has learned to use to satisfy her emotional needs—for some period of time. Finally, she can stand it no longer and eats everything in sight. The analogy is often made to breaking out of prison. The escaped dieter has to get in all the eating pleasure she can manage before she puts herself in jail once again. When a woman is no longer dieting and does not have to deprive herself of the foods she loves, the need to binge diminishes. There is no longer a feeling of "eat it all now, because tomorrow (or Monday or next month) it's back on the diet."

There will be those of you who, for various reasons (medical or otherwise), will choose to continue dieting. That is all right. You will still find much in this chapter which may help you to eat less compulsively. You should use my ideas in ways which fit into *your* needs and lifestyles. You must take from this chapter the concepts that appeal to you and apply them in your own way to your diet. For instance, some of the exercises on eating awareness teach you to discriminate desires for food textures and temperatures. At one meal, you may yearn for a crunchy, cold food, while at another the desire may be for warmth or smoothness. Within the context of your specific diet, these desires can usually be met, with the result that you will feel more satisfied with your meal. If, for example, you are feeling angry one afternoon and have a need for a food to bite down on, to release some of the tension, all the cottage cheese in the world (or ice cream, for that matter) will not satisfy your "hunger." On the other hand, the addition of a few crunchy carrots may transform the meal into a most agreeable one—satisfying both the requirements of your diet and your emotional need.

The exercises presented here do not constitute a new set of rules or a diet program. Rather, the exercises are experiments which provide you with new information and awareness.

It is my hope that you will allow yourself, at least for now, complete freedom with food. No food is to be forbidden or shunned as a high calorie or junk food. There are no "good" foods or "bad" foods. Rather than judging a food, observe your body's reaction to it. If the food is not right for *you*, your body will let you know. This is the time of learning all about your eating behavior. What does hunger feel like to you? Observe. There are many gradations of fullness, ranging from "no longer feeling hunger pangs" to "so stuffed I feel sick." What are these gradations? Experiment. Your body has so much to tell you if you let it—if you suspend judgment and listen. It may be difficult at first to envision living without strict rules and limitations on your eating, but you can take each step as slowly as you like. At times you may feel adrift at sea, floundering, without a strict set of rules specifying proper eating behavior. Yet, out of this confusion will emerge an inner direction, a sense that you know best what you need and that you can take care of yourself.

I cannot overemphasize the importance of *nonjudgmental* observation in effecting changes in your eating behavior. It probably feels as though you must hate yourself for overeating in order to stop; yet self-hate or disgust is actually a poor motivater. In fact, the bad feelings generated by self-hate often cause the compulsive eater to turn to more food for relief.

Several years ago, Timothy Gallwey brought to the public an exciting new approach to learning based on nonjudgmental awareness in his book, *The Inner Game of Tennis*. He writes of a natural learning process which unfolds if you allow it to. Though he was referring to tennis in his book, many of the concepts can be helpful to you as you begin to examine your eating behaviors in a new way. For instance, he writes, "The first inner skill to be developed in the Inner Game is that of nonjudgmental awareness. When we 'unlearn' judgment we discover, usually with some surprise, that we don't need the motivation of a reformer to change our 'bad' habits. There is a more natural process of learning and performing waiting to be discovered. It is waiting to show what it can do when allowed to operate without interference from the conscious strivings of the judgmental ego-mind."[3]

"How could removing the judgments help?" you might ask. "It would seem that if I stop telling myself it's bad to eat certain foods, if I don't get angry at myself for overeating, I'll just keep getting fatter and fatter." Yet, when you stop to think about it, ultimately the negative self-judgments have not solved your eating problem, nor have they even helped you to control it. Often they lead you to another binge to assuage your bad feelings; in addition, these negative judgments form a noisy confusion in your mind which keeps you from hearing your body's response to your eating. Compulsive eaters are often so busy hating themselves for overeating and eating even more in response that they are not able to make use of the feedback their bodies are sending in response to the food. In my compulsive eating days I could eat a half-gallon of ice cream with no trouble, but since I have learned to tune into my body's inner signals, I become overly full after as little as one cup. At first, I began to wonder how I had been able to stuff so much food in my stomach without becoming ill; yet now I realize that I was so busy obsessing about how horrible I was for having so little willpower and eating so much food that I never stopped to feel how very full I really was. The feedback was there. I was just not picking it up. Once you get in touch with these inner bodily sensations you can never eat as much again.

I have said that diets are the prescriptions from others as to what, when, and how you should eat. Yet, even when not dieting, compulsive eaters are outer-directed in their eating behavior. In many experiments it has been demonstrated that overweight people are affected by external stimuli—sights, sounds, smells of food—in deciding when and what to eat. The signal to eat is not coming from an inner sensation, but from outside the person. You might think about how often you have eaten a bowl of potato chips because someone put it down in front of you, or stopped in a bakery because of the aroma of freshly baked goods. Behavior modification approaches, mindful of this problem for the overeater, recommend arranging the environment so that such external stimuli will not be present or at least their presence will be minimized. For instance, one is to eat only at specified times and places or food is to be placed in cabinets where it will not be seen. Obviously, the externals cannot always be under your control. Some one may plant that bowl of potato chips right in front of you some day. Therefore, the approach presented here is aimed not at controlling these external stimuli, but on turning your focus of attention inward and teaching you to eat primarily out of bodily need.

During this portion of your inner journey I would like you to suspend temporarily any efforts to lose weight. I realize that it is almost impossible for a compulsive eater to conceive of living even one day without striving for that ultimate goal of thinness. However, trying to lose weight at the same time you are learning a new way of eating, tends to create pressure and may prevent you from learning effectively. In fact during the initial stages of observation, it is best not to *change* your eating behavior at all. Just observe. For those of you already on a diet, it is okay to continue, but try to view this portion of your inner journey as a time to maintain (not necessarily lose) weight. It may even be helpful for you to experience a period of time in which you are neither gaining nor losing weight. It will probably be the first time. Most compulsive eaters have had little experience maintaining a steady weight—usually they are either on the way up or on the way down. This period of maintaining a steady weight will be a good preparation for life as a thin person who is no longer dieting.

The first step in this process will include a period of observation of others' eating patterns, as well as your own food intake. I recommend beginning with a chart of all the foods you eat for an entire week, or even longer if possible. The purpose of this chart is not to limit your eating, but to provide you instead with information as to what you eat, when, and under what conditions.

Food eaten	Where	Emotional State before eating	Degree of hunger	How you feel after eating emotionally	How you feel after eating physically
Comments					

Now that you have begun examining your own eating patterns, I would like you to begin observing other people's eating behavior. Watch your family members, your friends, even strangers in restaurants. Observe compulsive eaters, compulsive dieters, naturally thin people, children. Keep the following questions in mind for each person you observe:

1) How is this person eating? quickly, gobbling down the food, or slowly with careful attention to each bite?

2) Does this person pause between bites, or does one mouthful follow the other?
3) What is this person's emotional state? nervous? calm? joyful? distracted? How does his/her eating reflect this state?
4) Does this person seem comfortable around food?
5) Is there anything left over on this person's plate when he or she is through?

There is much to learn from the observation of others' eating behaviors. Did you notice, for example, that naturally thin people (those who are not constantly dieting) will stop eating as soon as they feel full, no matter how much is left on their plates? Or did you notice how little investment they may have had in their food, pausing to chat a bit between bites? If possible, it would help to talk to a woman whom you have identified as a naturally thin person, and ask her questions about how she eats and how she deals with problems in her life without turning to food.

Now let us explore the experience of hunger. Hunger has both physical and psychological components and evokes different emotional responses in each person. The signal to eat in a compulsive eater, however, has little to do with true physical hunger, as you may have learned from your food chart. Such variables as time, place, and emotional state play a larger part than any inner physical sensations. It would be unrealistic to expect a person in our culture to disregard totally the factors of time, place, and emotion in determining when to eat, but the closer you can come to feeding yourself out of real physical need, the more true to yourself you become — and the more "in tune."

For the compulsive eater the emotions, more than any other factor, contribute to the problem of eating when the body is not in need of nourishment. As we discussed earlier, the compulsive eater turns to food when she is happy or sad, bored or excited, fearful or calm, up or down. She has given food the power to deal with these emotions. As we have seen, all emotions have a physical component in the body, and the problem lies in the compulsive eater's inability to differentiate between the inner sensations of hunger, anger, fear, or excitation. For example, each time a woman fails to assert herself—saying "yes" when she meant "no" or allowing herself to be insulted—there may be a little twinge in the body. Very often this sensation is even experienced in the stomach as a sort of dropping feeling. The compulsive eater wrongly interprets this sensation as hunger and proceeds to eat. (You must remember that in many cases this entire process is only partly conscious.) Working through the preceding chapters will have prepared you to differentiate various internal sensations. By now you will have become aware of some of your fears of being "in touch" with your body's physical and psychological states. Now your work should focus on recognizing hunger signals and learning to respond to them appropriately.

Though you may have made progress in getting "in touch" with your body's internal messages, you may still have reservations about trusting yourself to recognize true hunger and respond appropriately. We have already discovered how women, especially those who have dieted strenuously, have been taught to distrust their bodies' messages. Susie Orbach provides an interesting analogy which may help you get beyond your initial distrust. She points out that a person generally reacts automatically to a full bladder. "Again," she writes, "most people will grow up with a confidence about knowing how to follow the signals that they need to urinate and the amount will vary considerably. Sometimes, there will be a great deal of pressure on the bladder, sometimes less, but the information that one needs relief will become available quite obviously."[4] You have the ability to perceive and react to physical hunger in the same manner.

Perhaps you lack trust because you have never really felt hunger. Many of my patients have reported such a reaction. They eat so much and so often that the physical sensations of hunger never have a chance to appear. For those of you in this position, it may be a little uncomfortable at first to wait until you feel hungry before you eat, but as the newness of the feeling wears off, hunger soon becomes like an old friend gently reminding you it is time to eat.

Some of you may fear hunger because you *have* known it. Some of my patients, victims of the Holocaust, have terrible associations with hunger: memories of near-starvation and bellies crying out to be fed. Those of you who fear hunger for this or similar reasons may have to take this portion of your journey especially slowly. Be aware that unpleasant memories may arise at this time, and do not try to fight them. These feelings will diminish eventually when you truly trust that your hunger now is not the starvation of the past. Those patients I have worked with who feared letting themselves get hungry have all overcome this difficulty without extreme anxiety.

"How do I go about learning to distinguish the sensations of physical hunger from those of other bodily states?" you may ask at this point. True, physical hunger is felt by most people as a grumbling, gnawing feeling in the stomach, sometimes accompanied by a slight emptiness too. Feelings of hunger also tend to come and go, returning each time with a slightly greater intensity. For me these early sensations are not at all uncomfortable, but pleasant reminders that my body is ready for a meal. If these initial messages are ignored for some time, however, stronger, definitely unpleasant messages are sent out: headaches, faintness, fatigue.

At first it may be difficult deciding whether the sensation you are feeling in your mouth or stomach is real or psychological hunger, but eventually you will learn to distinguish. Although the goal toward which you are striving is to eat only out of physical need, at the beginning much of your eating will still be to satisfy emotional needs. That is okay for now, since you have no way to satisfy these needs other than through food. As you begin to take the power back from food, you will turn to eating less and less to meet emotional needs.

In order to learn more about how you experience hunger, I would like you to again observe your eating behavior, this time focusing on the physical sensations of hunger. The following questions will help you:

Hunger Awareness Exercise

1) How do I know I am hungry? How does my body let me know it needs food? What are the physical sensations which signal

hunger? Is there a grumbling, a gnawing, or an emptiness in my stomach? Are the physical sensations which make me feel like eating the same as those I have identified as hunger?
2) How often do I get hungry during the day? Once? Twice? Many times? Does the number of times I feel hungry vary from day to day? If I eat breakfast, how many hours does it take before I feel hungry again? Do different foods influence how soon I feel hungry again after breakfast? For instance, a meal of toast and jam may leave some people starving after only two hours, while eggs and a bran muffin may satiate their hunger for hours.
3) Does eating certain foods make me hungrier for more?
4) Is my first signal of hunger a headache or a feeling of lightheadedness? If so, either you are hypoglycemic or else you are missing earlier, more subtle signals your body is sending.
5) How do I react to the physical sensations of hunger? Are the sensations of hunger pleasurable or uncomfortable? Am I excited about the prospect of eating? Do I have a twinge of fear? What is this fear about? Complete the sentence: "If I feel hungry then . . ." or, "If I let myself feel hungry then. . . ."

Whether hunger stems from physical or psychological sources, it is accompanied by certain bodily sensations that provide information about what type of food is needed. Leonard and Lillian Pearson, in their book, *The Psychologist's Eat-Anything Diet*, have identified four areas of the body in which these sensations are usually felt.[5]

Stomach Hunger

Though sensations in this area are usually a sign of true physical hunger, sometimes there is also a disturbing feeling in the pit of the stomach, a kind of hole that needs to be filled up quickly. This kind of hunger often produces a binge. Yet just a little of the right food will often do the trick. The Pearsons state that the kinds of foods which usually satisfy this type of hunger are bulky, warm, filling foods, often starches—spaghetti, a warm, soft dinner roll, thick soups—exactly the type of foods most dieters avoid. Instead of turning to the food which is needed to quell the hunger, the dieter chooses "low calorie" alternatives—cottage cheese or carrots, for example—but because these foods do not satisfy, will not fill up that empty pit, more and more food is consumed. Eventually the compulsive eater has worked her way to a binge that does not end until the stomach aches from fullness. A small bowl of hot, thick soup may have provided fewer calories than the collection of food actually eaten, and certainly would have created much more satisfaction.

Throat and Mouth Hunger

Hunger can also be experienced in the back of the throat and in the mouth. Though the Pearsons grouped these two areas together, I prefer to deal with them separately.

The sensations of mouth hunger are probably the most familiar to the compulsive eater. There is a tingling, an emptiness inside the mouth, accompanied by a compulsion to get something into the mouth immediately. Often one experiences a desire for just the taste of something, usually something sweet or cool. The Pearsons point out that people often go through an entire meal just to get to the dessert. If you are one of these people, you are consuming a lot of extra food (and calories, if you still think in those terms) just so you will be able to have the sweet food you really crave. It was quite a revelation to me when I realized I could go to a restaurant and order only a Caesar salad and dessert and be supremely satisfied. When I am in tune with my body and aware of my hunger for a sweet taste, even hot rolls with butter do not appeal to me. It takes no will power to turn them down, when I know I will soon be having exactly the right food to satisfy my mouth hunger. The rolls would merely *fill me up* at such a time. The dessert will *satisfy*. The mouth hunger may also call for a particular type of seasoning or flavor: a sharp, tangy Cheddar or a mild Havarti with dill, for example.

Throat hunger can be felt as a tightness or dryness at the back of the throat. Like the sensations of mouth hunger, these sensations are usually satisfied with something cool—often a cold beverage. One of my patients discovered that sucking on an ice cube would quell this hunger, while another was satisfied with cool mineral water. The slight carbonation of this water produced a most satisfying sensation at the back of the throat.

Gum and Teeth Hunger

Have you ever had the desire just to sink your teeth into something soft and chewy? This is a form of teeth hunger, a hunger which cannot be satisfied by just any food. All the ice cream and cake in the world will leave you unfulfilled, if you are experiencing this need to chew. Actually, teeth and gum hunger can be expressed as a desire for soft chewy foods (bagels, soft rolls, gum) or hard crunchy foods (carrots, pretzels, or nuts, for example). This kind of hunger is often experienced as a dull ache or tingling in the teeth and gums. Other foods which satisfy this hunger are steaks, corn, chicken (with bones intact), potato chips, and celery.

Tongue and Lip Hunger

Foods to lick or suck satisfy this type of hunger. Ice cream cones are a favorite choice, because they allow both licking and sucking pleasure. The Pearsons suggest sucking cheese (a marvelous experience if you like cheese) or drinking a beverage through a straw. You might enjoy carrots or celery covered with a tangy, creamy dip, licking off the dip as you go along.

Once you have located the source of your hunger it is easier to identify foods that will satisfy. Let us explore the choice of foods further. How do you decide which food will best satisfy your hunger at any given moment? The Pearsons' approach may prove helpful. Early in their book they introduce the concept of humming and beckoning foods. Foods that "hum" are those which satisfy an inner craving. If you experience a sudden craving for a particular food, a craving that arises spontaneously without your even having seen the food, you are familiar with a food that "hums." On the other hand, the food you eat just because it is there is "beckoning." You pass the bakery, smell the sweet aroma of freshly baked bread, and decide to buy some. Some one places a bowl of nuts in front of you and you begin to eat them. Your child leaves some food over on her plate and you eat it, almost unconsciously, as you clear away the dishes. These foods were "beckoning." You had no inner need to eat them, you did not yearn for them. You saw them, they called out to you, and you ate them.

The goal is to eat foods which "hum" as often as possible. These foods will truly satisfy your hunger, and it will probably not take much food to do so. On the other hand, you may not feel satisfied with even a large amount of a "beckoning" food. For example, a crunchy chicken salad with lots of mayonnaise may be "humming" to you one day, but it feels like too much trouble to make the salad or go out for one, so you grab the coffee cake on the counter and cut off a piece, and another and another. Half the cake may be gone, but you are still not satisfied. Yet a small portion of the chicken salad may have left you satisfied for hours. Even if your portion is not small, it is likely to add up to fewer calories than half a cake. Again, I refer to the calorie counts not to encourage keeping account of calories, but just to give you an idea of how eating the foods which "hum" leads to less food consumption and eventually to weight loss.

At this point, I think it is important to explain my views on good and bad food, fattening and nonfattening food. Unless you must diet for medical or strong emotional reasons, I suggest that you allow yourself complete freedom in your choice of foods. No food is good or bad, fattening or slimming in itself. A food is only right or wrong for *you*. The exercises in this chapter will help you determine which foods best satisfy your own physical and emotional needs. One overweight woman may have an emotional and physical makeup which makes her especially sensitive to refined sugars. Foods containing such sugars create adverse reactions in her nervous system and lead her to crave more. She may have also learned early in childhood to turn to sweets as a reward for hardship. Another overweight woman may be little affected by the same foods—she can take them or leave them, consuming small amounts of sugary foods only occasionally. It does not help to label the sugar "bad." Such labeling certainly will not stop the first woman from consuming sweets. In fact, eating a "bad" food is likely to engender guilt in such a person—and such guilt only leads her to eat more. Furthermore, what is "bad" for one woman is not so for another.

The following food awareness exercise will help you determine which foods are "humming" when you are hungry:

Food Awareness Exercise

Wait until you feel hungry, in order to try this exercise. The following steps will help you determine what food will satisfy that hunger. It is best to isolate yourself from food while you are making your decision, so that your choice comes from inner need, rather than from a food that "beckons."

1. Sit for a minute and concentrate on the sensations of hunger. Where in your body do you feel these feelings? Mouth? Throat? Lips? Tongue? Teeth? Stomach? The sensations may originate from two or even more locations at the same time. How strong are these sensations?
2. Close your eyes, if possible, and imagine a food coming to mind—a food that will satisfy your hunger. It may take a few moments at first to envision a food, but with practice this process will become second nature. Some day you will just *know* what you want without conscious thought, but during this period of learning a conscious effort must be made.
3. If no food arises spontaneously, ask yourself some questions to narrow down the choices. Do I want something smooth or crunchy? Hot or cold? Spicy or bland? Juicy or dry and crisp? Keep in mind the areas of your body that are feeling the hunger. For example, you may be feeling sensations in your mouth and stomach. First, ask, "What kind of taste is my mouth looking for?" The answer may be spicy, in this instance. Next, ask, "What kind of food will satisfy these feelings in my stomach?" The answer might be something hot and creamy and starchy. "Macaroni with a thick, tangy Cheddar sauce" might immediately come to mind. If you can almost smell the aroma and taste its sharp, creamy flavor, then you know this food is right for you. It is humming.

It may be that the food which is "humming" is not easily or readily available. In that case, try to find another food that will satisfy the sensations of hunger or select a close approximation of your first choice. Usually, however, the food that comes to mind is obtainable, though at times it may take a little effort on your part to prepare or buy it. Make an effort to eat the food that "hums," even if you have to work hard to get it. If you would go out of your way to prepare a special dish for someone you love, why not do so for yourself? You will be telling yourself, "I'm worthy of extra attention. I can take care of my food needs and satisfy my hunger." Remember, too, it will take a lot less of the right food to satisfy yourself.

4. When you think you have identified the food that best satisfies your hunger, imagine yourself eating. What will it taste like in your mouth? Imagine its temperature, its texture. How will it feel going down? In your stomach? If the food feels like it will satisfy the hunger, then you can be sure you have picked the right food. If something does not feel quite right, then maybe you have not identified *exactly* what you want. Let us look at another example. You know that your hunger calls for something smooth and creamy — ice cream, perhaps — but when you imagine yourself eating the ice cream, you do not feel quite satisfied. It is too cold. So you think again. "Smooth and creamy, not too cold — ricotta cheese, whipped in the blender with just a bit of honey and vanilla!" You imagine eating the ricotta and it feels just right. Go ahead and enjoy!

Let me repeat that at first the process of choosing the best food will seem complicated and lengthy. "I want to learn to think about food less, not *more*," you may exclaim; but learning to choose the foods which best satisfy your physical and emotional needs is like any other learned behavior. It takes work and practice at the beginning, and eventually the behavior becomes second nature. Remember learning to drive a car or ride a bike. Think of a new skill you have acquired. Even though your body knows without any training what kinds of foods it needs, you have become so out of touch with the messages, you have to *learn* to listen to them all over again. This will take some time. Just be patient.

One Bowl by Don Gerrard offers another way to determine what foods will satisfy. Rather than labeling foods as either good/bad or legal/illegal, he distinguishes between those which are harmonious with the body and those which are disruptive to it. "All this is eating," he writes. "It is like a symphony—many elements must come together in harmony. When they do, music is made and one is nourished. When they don't the result is noise and discomfort." He writes further, "You will lose weight and gain energy as you learn to increase the harmony in your internal food symphony."[6] Those foods which are disruptive or discordant create digestive upsets and waste, or fat. Harmonious foods leave you feeling good both physically and emotionally.

How can you tell which foods are harmonious and which disruptive? Your body will tell you. Just as you had to learn your body's signals for hunger, now you must concentrate on discerning the myriad messages your body sends as you eat a meal. The next two exercises aim at increasing your awareness.

Eating Awareness Exercise I—Tasting

I suggest taping this exercise or having someone read it to you as you eat the food. Gerrard recommends eating only one food at a sitting, so as to concentrate on that food alone and how it makes you feel. Eating only one food at a time will enable you to determine which foods are harmonious and which are disruptive to your body. I realize that it is not usually feasible to eat this way, but for the purposes of this exercise try to focus on only one food at a time.

Once you have chosen a food that will satisfy your body's hunger, you are ready to eat.

1. Sit for a moment and look at the food you have chosen. What is its color? texture? temperature? Prepare yourself for the pleasurable eating experience to come. Smell the food. Does the aroma appeal to you? Does it whet your appetite? Do you find smelling the food pleasurable? offensive?
2. Now take one bite of the food. Feel its texture and experience its flavor. Focus your full attention on the feel of this food in your mouth. Swallow. How does it feel going down? Does this first bite affect the sensations of hunger?
3. Try another bite and another, each time repeating the process described in Step 2. How does it feel to focus full attention on

the process of eating? Does it feel uncomfortable? Pleasurable? Do you feel like doing something else while you eat? If so, what do you think this feeling is about? Guilt over the sensual pleasure you are allowing yourself? Guilt over your judgments of the value or calorie count of the food? Are you merely in the habit of doing something else while you eat? The more you can focus all your attention on what is taking place inside you as you eat, the easier it will be to listen to and interpret your body's messages. Reading, talking or watching television merely distracts you from this internal focusing. Keep in mind that you won't always have to pay such careful attention to your eating, but for this period of learning it is helpful to concentrate as often as possible on the process of eating without external distraction.
4. When you have finished your meal spend a few minutes trying to determine your body's reaction to the food you have just eaten. How do you feel? full? satisfied? bloated? uncomfortable? Do not judge, just observe.
5. A half hour or an hour later your body will still be sending messages as to its reaction to the meal. Check out these messages. What is your body trying to tell you?
    — Is there any feeling of discomfort? If so, where?
    — Do you feel any kind of pain? Heartburn?
    — Do you feel light and comfortable, or bloated and nervous?
    — Are there any unusual physical or emotional reactions to the food? One patient of mine discovered that whenever she ate bananas, she experienced extreme sleepiness an hour later. Another found chocolate made her nervous presumably due to a sensitivity to the caffeine it contains.

Discussion of Eating Awareness Exercise I

Most compulsive eaters will experience some difficulty in eating slowly. Though some of the difficulty can be attributed to breaking a lifelong habit of rapid eating, other factors may be even more important. Beth's experience can illustrate this point. Despite frequent attempts she was unable to slow down her eating; in fact, she became aware she was virtually swallowing large chunks of food unchewed at a rapid pace. Beth realized eating was not the pleasurable experience she had thought it was, but a somewhat tense, hurried experience. Since she was still unable to slow down and enjoy her food despite her awareness of the problem, Beth began to suspect there was some reason why she needed to eat quickly. "What am I afraid of? What wouldn't I *like* about eating slowly? What wouldn't feel right about it?" These were some of the questions she grappled with. The answers were surprising. She realized first of all that there was a quality to her style of eating which paralleled her approach to living. "I 'swallowed whole' chunks of life the way I was swallowing whole chunks of food. I was unable to slow down and digest life's experiences for fear that if I were to relax my hold on myself, I'd be overwhelmed with experiences. I'd just collapse." Similarly, if she slowed down and began to taste the food she was eating, Beth feared she might be overwhelmed with sensations ("I might collapse"). Learning to relax was her real task, and eating slowly would follow naturally. Once she had determined why she was unable to slow down her eating, Beth was able to do something about it.

Some of you may have had trouble eating slowly because it felt like you would not get to eat your "share." This problem is true for women who live in or grew up in homes where everyone ate quickly, and a slow eater would find all the food gone before she had had enough. The solution to such a problem is to have a portion set aside for yourself which is yours alone, whether you choose to eat all of it at once or to save some of it for later. It is important to make sure that your food will always be available to you. If you know it will always be there, the need to eat it all quickly will diminish.

Foods which leave you feeling good in body and mind are "harmonious" foods. Those which make you feel uncomfortable or uneasy are disruptive to your well-being. The idea, according to Gerrard, is to eat foods which are harmonious for you and avoid disruptive foods. What is harmonious to one person will make another ill, so you can see how labeling of foods as "good" and "bad" is inadequate and even erroneous. You must learn which foods are harmonious and which are disruptive for you alone. Once you realize that a particular food has a bad effect on your body, you will *tend* not to want to eat it. I emphasize "tend" because it is not my intent or my expectation that you will never eat that food. To say "don't eat disruptive foods" is to set you up with a new diet rule and one you would soon want to break. If you still want to eat a food which you have found to be disruptive in the past, go ahead. My experience shows that *as long as you truly feel the freedom to eat it*, you will tend to want to avoid the food which makes you feel uncomfortable.

Your body's reactions to food may sometimes surprise you. I had always believed I had an "iron stomach," but much to my surprise I discovered one day, by paying careful attention to my body's internal signals, that I could not easily digest a bagel. Hours after eating one I still was feeling heaviness and fullness in my stomach—a nagging discomfort of which I had never before been aware. Once I became aware of what the bagels were doing to my sense of well-being, my desire to eat them diminished greatly. No will power nor effort was required. I just did not want to eat them because of how they made me feel.

What amazed me about this discovery was that I had eaten bagels all my life and had never realized they made me feel sick. How could I have missed for so many years what now seemed such loud messages of protest from my body? The difference, I believe, is that in the past I was so out of touch with my body's internal signals that these messages did not register in my conscious mind.

Such is the case for all compulsive eaters. The messages are there, you just have to learn to read them. Once you begin to pay attention, however, you will be amazed at what your body has to say and how strong these bodily sensations can feel. As I mentioned earlier, I still marvel at my ability during my compulsive eating days to down a half-gallon of ice cream in one sitting with no apparent ill effects. Now a small portion is all I can handle—more makes me feel stuffed, and an entire half-gallon would make me quite ill. Yet I am the same person. All that has changed is my ability to listen to my body's reactions to food. The signals feel more intense now that I am aware of them but they have always been there. Once you become aware of them you will not ever lose this sensitivity again. Almost every woman I have worked with has experienced this reaction. Even the capacity to binge diminishes. Someone who was capable of eating a bag of cookies finds she now "binges" on five or six. Eventually the binges disappear altogether.

Gerrard goes even further in his book, *One Bowl*, to help you learn to differentiate between even more subtle sensations indicating your body's reaction to a food "than those commonly recognized as digestive upset."[7] He recommends trying to discern such sensations as

- an area of emptiness
- a movement as a result of temperature changes
- an area of sound
- a sharp, one-time sound[8]

I must confess that in all my years of learning to discern my bodily sensations, I have yet to fine-tune my awareness to such a degree of sensitivity, but I keep trying.

Your newly emerging sensitivity will also be helpful in the next part of your journey of self-discovery—determining when you have had enough to eat. Just as your body sends messages about specific foods, it also broadcasts constant messages indicating degrees of fullness. The degree of fullness can range from "no longer feeling hunger pangs" to "so stuffed I feel ill." The following exercise will help you learn to differentiate among these various states of fullness.

Eating Awareness Exercise II—Fullness

This exercise is similar to the previous one, but the focus of attention will be only those body sensations which signal that you have had enough to eat. Let me remind you again that you will not always have to pay such careful attention to your eating, but in order to learn it you must expend effort and concentration. After a while the process of determining when you have had enough to eat will take little conscious thought or effort.

1. Begin eating your food with careful attention to taste and texture.
2. After each bite check out its effect on your hunger. What are

you feeling in your stomach? After several bites you should be able to discern some change in the state of your hunger. Each additional bite will make some degree of change, however small. In order to give your body time to adjust to the intake of food, it is important to eat slowly and chew as thoroughly as possible. I am not recommending that you eat slowly as a way of cutting down your food intake, as many diet programs suggest, but as a way of giving your body the time it needs to react to the food it is receiving and to send out the appropriate messages in response. Gobbling down large chunks of undigested food will only serve to confuse your body, and it is likely that you will eat well past the point of fullness before your body has had time to send its message.

3. After eating some portion of your meal—half a sandwich, for example—get up from the table and go to another room where you will not see the food. It is difficult to tune into your internal messages of fullness while you are sitting in front of an array of food. The food "beckons" and the compulsive eater continues eating, paying less and less attention to the internal signals. leaving the room is not intended as a punishment, nor is it a trick to get you to stop eating. I recommend leaving the room for the purposes of this exercise, so that you will not be distracted in your attempts to listen to your body. Now turn your attention inside your body. Ask yourself these questions:

—What are you feeling? Is your stomach full? If so, how would you feel if you were to stop eating now?

—Are you still hungry? Where do you feel the hunger? mouth? throat? stomach?

—If you are still hungry, will the food you have been eating satisfy that hunger or do you want something else? What food will satisfy that hunger?

4. If you have determined you are no longer hungry you might try going back into the kitchen and putting away the rest of the food. How does this make you feel? good? fearful? deprived? If you feel that you *must* continue eating, though you are no longer hungry, go ahead. Do not judge yourself but be aware of the signals your body is sending as you continue your meal.

5. If you are still hungry, then by all means eat. As you eat, continue to monitor your body's signals.

Discussion of Eating Awareness Exercise II

Some of my patients quickly learn to distinguish the inner sensations which signal fullness, yet find it almost impossible to act on their knowledge—to stop when they feel comfortably full. Why is this? Some are disturbed to discover just how little food it takes to fill them up. "When I did this exercise," one patient exclaimed, "it suddenly struck me that if I kept on listening to what my body was telling me, I'd start eating less and less food. It almost feels like I'll be depriving myself—of quantity, I guess. It's scary to know that I can eat so little and be satisfied. I also realized that I *could* lose weight without dieting, simply by following my body's instructions." Sometimes a woman, despite such a realization, is not yet ready to take the step to lose weight, so she chooses (at least unconsciously) to disregard her body's signals and keep on eating past the point of fullness.

In other instances, a compulsive eater may not only disregard her body's messages, but tune them out entirely, to eat herself into oblivion. She does not even feel her body's urgent request to stop eating, because she has shut out all internal sensations from her consciousness. Usually this will happen when she wants to numb herself.

The next exercise will help you learn even more about your eating needs. It is adapted from an eating awareness exercise presented in *The Psychologist's Eat-Anything Diet*, and might be especially enjoyable. At the very least, you will have a strong reaction to the exercise. This exercise is best done with chocolate kisses, but if you are unable to eat chocolate for medical reasons, you may substitute some cheese.

The Chocolate Kiss Exercise

Unwrap one chocolate kiss. . . . Smell it. . . . How does the chocolate smell to you? . . . How often do you let yourself smell your food?

Now rub the chocolate over your lips. . . . Experience the sensations this creates for you. . . . And, if you have not already done so, lick your lips for your first taste of this chocolate. . . . Smell the chocolate again. The moistened chocolate may smell different to you now.

Now bite off a small piece of the kiss—about half. Put the other half down in its wrapper. Do not chew it yet, but place it between your tongue and your palate (the roof of your mouth). . . . Keeping the kiss pressed against the roof of your mouth, slowly rub your tongue over the chocolate. . . . Now put the chocolate under your tongue. . . . Begin to move it around your mouth . . . between your upper teeth and lips . . . between your cheek and teeth . . . sliding it around to the other cheek. . . . Slowly, sensuously, roll the chocolate around your mouth until it is all gone.

Now put the next half in your mouth—placing it again between your tongue and the roof of your mouth. . . . This time, as the kiss warms up and starts to melt, slowly suck on it, extracting the essence. . . . Move the chocolate around your mouth, learning as much as you can about where the chocolate feels best in your mouth. . . . How does it taste on your tongue? Which places on your tongue are the most sensitive to its taste? . . . How does the chocolate feel on your gums? Under your tongue? . . . Experience this chocolate kiss to its fullest. . . . When you have finished the kiss, run your tongue over your teeth . . . your gums . . . your cheeks . . . to pick up every last taste of the chocolate.

Now, unwrap a second chocolate kiss and chew it up as fast as you can. . . . Compare your experience with this kiss to the first one.

Discussion of Chocolate Kiss Exercise

Some of you may have enjoyed this exercise immeasurably; others may have disliked the chocolate exercise, because they did not like the sensation of chocolate covering their teeth or because they did not like that particular chocolate. The reactions to this exercise are varied, and it will be helpful to discuss each possibility separately.

The most common reaction is "I can't believe it took me five minutes to eat two chocolate kisses. Usually I'd be halfway through the bag by now." Not only does this exercise help you to slow down your eating, but you may begin to realize how much pleasure you can get from just a small amount of food. Usually a compulsive eater swallows down her chocolate so quickly she barely tastes what she is eating. It may amaze you to learn how much flavor there is in a little chocolate kiss when all attention is focused on getting full satisfaction from it. The lack of guilt about eating also contributes to the satisfaction from it. Constant negative judgments about the food one is eating distracts one from concentrating on its taste. Contrary to popular notions, guilt over eating can actually *increase* consumption. Typically, the compulsive eater, having gone off her diet and consumed some quantity of "forbidden" food, feels guilty. "How could I have done this? I'm a pig. I can't even control myself." Her guilt, however, only serves to make her feel bad, and how does a compulsive eater respond to feeling bad? She eats. She eats, feels more guilt, then eats again. Ironically, it is the absence of guilt which leads to less eating. Freed from the constant negative judgments about what she is eating, a woman can focus her attention on the taste of the food and derive full satisfaction.

It is likely that you felt little or no guilt about eating the chocolate in this exercise. Did you notice how the absence of guilt feelings contributed to your enjoyment? When you fully taste the food, it takes so little of it to satisfy.

Some of you, however, may have disliked the chocolate in the exercise—much to your surprise. "I thought I liked chocolate," some of my patients have said, "but the chocolate tasted so sweet—too sweet. It made me feel ill." Some women have discovered after doing this exercise that when they crave something sweet, an apple or banana will satisfy them without leaving a sickly sweet taste in the mouth. Others of you may have disliked the chocolate in this exercise for another reason—the chocolate was not good enough or was of the wrong kind. You may have discovered, as have others, that "when I eat chocolate, I want only the finest, the creamiest chocolate," or that "the taste of a bittersweet chocolate is much more satisfying to the palate." You will find, as you begin experimenting with food, that you become more and more discriminating, and of course, as you become more discriminating, you will find yourself turning away from junk—

satisfied with quality rather than quantity. In one of the six-session workshops I ran a few years ago, a woman came to me after the first session complaining about my approach to eating. "If you say I can eat whatever I want, all I will eat is ice cream—all day!" I assured her that it would be perfectly okay to eat ice cream every time she felt hungry, even if it meant eating *only* ice cream for as long as she craved it. At the end of the sixth session she announced, "I've discovered I don't like ice cream. I only like chocolate Haagen-Dazs (an expensive, creamy ice cream, available in some parts of the country), and if I can't have my chocolate Haagen-Dazs, I don't want ice cream at all." Having had complete freedom to eat ice cream without guilt, she was able to become so discriminating that only a particular brand appealed to her. Her ice cream consumption actually decreased during that period to less than she had consumed in all her years of dieting-bingeing.

I am sure you are wondering how you could allow yourself this kind of freedom with foods you love and not gain large amounts of weight. "Once I start eating ice cream (or cake or bread or whatever) I can't stop." Yet think for a moment. When foods are no longer forbidden, when you can have them any time you want, they begin to lose some of their specialness and their sinfulness. If you are never again going on a diet and you know you can always have another piece of that cake, later or tomorrow or next week, the need to finish the cake now diminishes. How many binges have had their origin in the thought that, "Tomorrow I'm going on a diet, so I'd better eat all I can tonight" or, "I blew my diet already today, so I might as well go ahead and eat"? Remember that you are working on the emotional meanings certain foods have for you and on taking back the power with which they have been endowed. After a while food will be just food to you, and it will take no great effort to eat a small portion of cake and stop when you are satisfied. For those of you who choose to diet, it will be a little more difficult to deal with "forbidden" foods, but I will discuss your problem later on in the chapter. For the time being, it might help to remember that feeling guilty over eating "forbidden" foods is not helpful, just accept it when it happens and go on from there.

Each time you eat a meal try to bring some measure of the effort and awareness you practiced in the eating awareness exercises to your own eating. I do not expect you to be aware of each bite and how it makes you feel, nor do I expect you to always leave the table midway through the family dinner, but the closer you can come to recreating the circumstances of the eating awareness exercises, the more intense will be your learning process. Some day you will be able to sit at a table filled with delicious foods and stop eating with no more thought or effort than you now give to brushing your teeth. Some day it will take no great effort to stop eating, but for now you will have to work at changing lifelong patterns of eating.

The remainder of this chapter will deal with questions you may have about this approach—questions which other women have asked me through the years. I hope the answers will enable you to integrate the awareness you have gained into your own lives.

How can I eat whatever I want and still lose weight?

This question will be discussed in full detail in the following chapter.

If you are in touch with your body's inner signals as to what food it needs and eat only as much food as it requires, your body weight will tend to normalize. You will eat only enough to support your body's functions, not enough though to support all your "extra" weight. Remember, when I say you can eat whatever you want, I do not mean you can eat with total abandon and still lose weight, but if you ate only ice cream all day, and *you ate only as much as it took to satisfy hunger*, you would lose weight.

It makes sense to me to eat only when I'm hungry, but I've got to be practical. My work hours are inflexible. I must eat at certain hours. How can I follow my body's signals?

Variations on this question are endless, but basically women want to know how they can fit such an ideal approach to eating into their own lifestyles. My answer may surprise you.

My approach to eating *is* an ideal to strive for but it is not an inflexible diet which must be followed to a tee. As much as possible, it is best to eat only when hungry, but at times you may have to adjust your eating somewhat to meet a schedule.

Let us look at how some of my patients have approached the problem. June worked in an office in which she was assigned a fixed lunch hour. Though she was often not hungry at that hour, she had to eat because she had no further access to food for the next six hours. When we looked for a solution to her problem, we discovered that there were two short coffee breaks at 11:00 and 3:00. If June ate a little something at 11:00 and "skipped lunch," she was usually hungry enough at 3:00 for another small meal. What she found she enjoyed most was sandwiches, eating half of the portion at 11:00, half at 3:00. June reserved the lunch hour for socializing with friends or relaxing. Another patient discovered that if she ate a little more than usual in the morning she did not get hungry again until after work. A third patient, a doctor, was able to keep food in her refrigerator in her office, and eat little bits at a time throughout the day. She might have a half cup of yogurt one time, a few bites of a sandwich between patients, and a cup of coffee with colleagues in the afternoon. As her schedule always varied, so did her eating.

From these examples, you can see that it is important to rethink the concept of "meals," a subject we will soon deal with. The more flexible and creative you can be, the better able you will be to fit this new eating approach into your life. There will be times that, despite all efforts, you are unable to match your food needs with your schedule. Sometimes you will be forced to eat at certain times, even though you are not hungry. That's okay. Just accept these limitations and relax. Perhaps at night or on weekends, you will have more freedom to choose when and what you eat. What I have presented is an ideal to strive for, and it does little good to hate yourself for not adhering to it perfectly. Remember, I am not proposing an inflexible diet, but an approach, a way of thinking about food.

What if everyone else is eating and I'm not hungry? What if I'm going out to lunch with others and I'm not hungry? What if my family is about to sit down to dinner and I'm not hungry?

All these questions are variations of the last one, and my answer is that you have to take each instance as it arises and make a decision about what is right for you at the time. For instance, you may have prepared a lovely meal for your family, but just do not feel like eating when it is time to sit down. First you have to be clear about what you want from the situation. Perhaps what you really want is the social contact. In that case, why eat? Why not just sit there and enjoy their company while they eat? On the other hand, you may feel if you just sat there, you would *not* enjoy their company, since your family meals are fraught with fights. Eating may be a way of putting some distance between yourself and what is going on with others at the table. If this is the case, perhaps you ought to rethink the situation. Eating is an important part of your life — a meal is a kind of self-giving and renewal. Ought you to be eating at a time of emotional tension? Do you really want to be there at all? Whatever your decision, perhaps your awareness of how your eating is functioning in this situation will prompt you to face the real issue — family strife. But if you still need to avoid the issue, must you use food as a means of doing so?

On the other hand, some may find that sitting down to a family meal is important in their lives — a kind of sharing and partaking in food *together*. If this is the case, you might want to eat just a little something, a salad or fruit, for example, to have a sense of sharing in the eating experience.

No matter what you choose to do, however, the key points are to be aware of what your needs are in the situation and to be flexible enough with your eating to meet these needs.

What if I'm hungry, but I don't know what to eat? Nothing hums.

If you feel real hunger and cannot discern what food will satisfy you, then just begin asking yourself questions. "Do I want something warm or cool? crunchy or soft? sweet or tart?" The answers to these questions will allow you to narrow down the choices and bring you closer to deciding what you would like. When you think you have identified the food, test it out by imagining yourself eating it. If it feels right, then go ahead and eat. If despite your questioning you still do not know what to eat, then just have a little something, a piece of cheese or a cracker to take the edge off your hunger, and wait until later to eat a meal.

What if I'm not physically hungry, but I feel the need to eat anyway?

If you need to eat for emotional reasons and cannot or do not want to think things through (such as determining what you are giving the food the power to do and whether you can accomplish it without food), then it is important to choose a food which will be most satisfying. For instance, in a fit of anger, you may tear into the kitchen and begin eating everything you find. Perhaps it would be more effective to ask yourself what food will give you the *most* satisfaction. Perhaps you would like to crunch down on thick carrots or crisp crackers. Why waste your time on the ice cream if it will not be effective in helping you discharge your anger? Certainly if you can zero in on the most effective food you will ultimately consume a lot less. Do not berate yourself for still having to use food to meet an emotional need. Just accept where you are. Change will come of its own some day, out of your very acceptance of where you are right now.

Sometimes I am aware that I'm full well before I've finished everything on my plate, but I can't leave the food over. I end up eating the rest of my food, even though I'm no longer hungry. What can I do about that?

The need to "clean your plate" is a common problem for women with compulsive eating problems. In order to decide what can be done about it, however, you first need to learn more about why you feel the need to finish everything on your plate. Next time you feel this urge, stop for a moment and ask yourself, "What would bother me about leaving over the rest of my food?" The answer to this question will provide you with clues as to how to approach the problem.

Betsy, for instance, felt a sense of deprivation in leaving over food that she felt was "rightfully hers." This feeling had its origin in the years of dieting, in which Betsy was allowed what was on her plate but no more, no less. "Feeling deprived on the diet, anyway, I felt I had to eat everything that was coming to me." The solution in this case was simple. Betsy first had to realize that she was no longer on a diet, and that the food would still be there later if she wanted it. Knowing that she could finish the food an hour later or three hours later or whenever she was hungry again made it easier for her to stop when full and put away the rest. Even those of you on a diet can look at meals this way. If you are "entitled" to all the food on your plate, but you are full half way through, why not put the rest away until later, when you are hungry again. Either way you will be consuming the same quantity.

Some of you may have difficulty leaving over food because of your early training not to waste food. There are two ways to view this problem. First of all, in many cases the food can be saved and eaten at another time. In a restaurant you can ask to have it wrapped up to take home. Even if it is not possible to save the food left over on your plate, the food is no more wasted if thrown out than if you eat it. If your body is signaling it has had enough, then you have taken in all the food it can use right now. Any extra food will be stored in your body as fat. The food will be just as wasted in your body as it would be if it were thrown out.

Some of you may have other reasons to finish your plate. Jana, a member of a rather large family, feared that if she did not eat her share at the table, then the food might not be there for her later. Even if she wrapped up her half sandwich and put it away somewhere else in the house, some one was likely to take it. The solution for Jana was to sit down with her family and explain that she was having a problem with food and that in order to get over the problem she needed to have food that was hers alone, to be eaten whenever she needed. Jana asked that food she left over and labeled be left untouched. Her family agreed.

What if I must diet? I have hypoglycemia (or diabetes or high blood pressure) and I must restrict my choice of foods. How can I still apply the principles you have shown me here?

Many of my patients are limited by diets required for medical reasons. What I suggest for such people is an emphasis on eating awareness with the actual food choices limited by the diet. For instance, at lunchtime a dieter can ask herself, "Do I want something hot or cold, chewy or smooth," and so on, and restrict the choices to those foods which are acceptable on her diet. A lot more satisfaction may be found in a hot broth with steamed vegetables than in a cold tuna plate, if the need is for warmth. More will be said on dieting per se in the next chapter.

What about nutrition?

I can best answer this question from a personal standpoint. I have always been and still am an avid reader of nutritional magazines and books of all kinds. Yet in the past, no matter what I had learned about the dangers of "junk food," when a binge occurred (and they so often did) I would nevertheless eat large quantities of such foods. No intellectual knowledge could successfully motivate me to change my eating habits, because my motivation to eat these foods came largely from unconscious needs. I required a period (which turned out to be several years) in which I could have the freedom to eat these foods—the cakes, candies, ice cream— without judgment. After a while ice cream and such lost some of its appeal, because it was no longer "forbidden" or "sinful." I had had my fill. Then, using my growing awareness of my body, I began to observe more closely the effects these foods had on me. The more aware I became of how they affected my functioning, the less I wanted to eat them.

At the same time I was working on the associations and the emotional attachments I had to sugary foods. Ice cream, for example, was a reward, a way of "sweetening up" my day. As I began to find new ways to meet these emotional needs, as I took the power back from the food, my desire for sugary foods further decreased. They had lost their magic. They had become *just foods*. Yet I continued to crave the taste of chocolate and other sugary foods in my mouth. Eventually, after much reading and reflecting, I decided that some of my desire for these foods might be coming from a *physical* dependence on refined sugar—a kind of addiction. It was at this point that I decided to give up foods with refined sugar entirely. After a week of strong withdrawal symptoms (headaches, malaise, nervousness) I found I no longer craved the sugar at all. Although I will never know if I had a physical addiction to sugar (in fact, a taste of sugar does not bring back the craving, as one would expect with a physical addiction), I know that I had to experience a period of time without it in order to get over my craving. In order to experiment as I did, though, I also needed all those years of permission to eat any food I craved without judgment.

As you can see, I evolved to a state of improved nutrition. No amount of will power could have made me stop eating sugar, though intellectually I knew how bad a diet of junk food could be for my body. If you just listen to your body and at the same time work on your emotional attachments to food, you too will move toward a diet which is healthy for you.

I must emphasize at this point the importance of finding a way of eating which is healthy for each individual. Years of reading different approaches to nutrition served only to confuse me, as it has others. Some books recommend high protein, others high carbohydrate, low protein. Some nutritional approaches state that all foods should be cooked, while others recommend raw foods. Some say milk is a good protein food, others refer to it as a poison, fit only for baby cows. All approaches claim their adherents are the healthiest, and they provide many case illustrations to prove it. I became more and more confused, until finally I realized that different people require different foods for optimum health. While one person will fare well on a macrobiotic diet consisting primarily of rice and some cooked vegetables, another will only feel healthy on a high protein diet with milk and meat. The only way to discover what was right for me was to follow my body's reactions to different foods as a guideline. I discovered, for instance, that I am one of those people who function best on a medium level protein diet with lots of raw vegetables and fruits. When I do not get enough protein, my body lets me know by its lowered resistance to infection.

Everyone is different. Everyone has her own nutritional needs. Look to your *body* to tell you what is right for you. I do not mean to imply, however, that your intellect ought not to be included in decisions about what is best for you. You might choose to stay away from foods with artificial dyes or preservatives, for example, because of what you have learned they can do to you. Your decisions about what food you eat ought to come from a combination of intellectual knowledge and careful attention to your body's messages. Mind and body combined will lead you to a way of eating most healthful for *you*.

six

The Power of Food

Look over the following statements. Do any of them sound familiar?

"When I'm depressed, I eat."
"As soon as I feel anxious I reach for the refrigerator."
"Sometimes I just can't stop eating, and I don't know why."
"When there's nothing to do at night I just eat—first cookies, then potato chips, then ice cream, then. . . ."
"Sometimes I diet all day, and then for some reason before I go to sleep, I eat just enough to blow my diet."

Any eating you do which is not specifically to satisfy physical hunger must be satisfying something else. Many compulsive eaters are aware that they use food to meet emotional needs—to pep them up, to calm them down, to give them something to do, to push down their anger. The list goes on and on. One woman told me she eats no matter what she is feeling or what happens. "I eat because I'm happy. I eat because I'm sad. I even eat because the traffic light turned red."

Let us take this reasoning one step further. Let us imagine for instance a woman who states, "I eat when I'm depressed." If you ask her why, she is likely to answer, "Because food makes me feel better." Yet, did she (or do *you*) ever stop to think *how* food makes

The Power of Food

one feel better? By what mechanism does food, as it enters your mouth, affect your body? The answer is, there is no such mechanism.[1] Food does not and cannot affect your mood or feelings when it first enters your mouth. When you eat you are not shooting up with heroin nor are you ingesting a tranquilizer. If you feel better (or calmer or peppier or happier or even upset) upon eating, it is not the food itself that made you feel that way. "Well, I know that when I'm depressed and I eat, I feel better, so if it isn't the food that makes me feel better, then what is it?" you may ask. The answer is "You."

It is your *belief* that food can make you feel better which affects you. This is known as the placebo effect. When a doctor gives you a placebo or sugar pill and tells you it will help cure your headaches, for example, your headaches are likely to be relieved. Yet the sugar pill, an inert substance, can not really be responsible for curing the headache. What happens is that in your belief that you would be helped by the pill, you have created certain substances in your brain that relieve pain. You attributed power to the pill to cure you, but it was really *you* who had the power all along.

Food is a placebo, often literally a sugar pill. You believe food will help you and so it feels like it does. You give the food the power to do things for you—but the power actually resides within you. If you feel better after you eat, it is because *you have done something to yourself to make you feel better and have attributed the power to the food.* Food has been endowed with magical properties.

This idea of the power of food is a difficult one to understand, let alone accept. Perhaps the two exercises which follow will help you discover more about how you have given power to food.

Power of Food Exercise I

1. Think of a situation in which you have been involved recently, one in which you are aware you were using food to meet some emotional need and felt the food had done something for you.
2. Think of how you were feeling both during and after eating. Did it seem that the food made you feel different?
3. Knowing as you do now that the food itself did not change the

way you felt, what *was* responsible for the change? What were you doing to yourself to bring about the change?

Discussion of Power of Food Exercise I

You may have to ponder these questions for quite some time before you can really understand what you are doing when you put food in your mouth. A few examples of how other women have dealt with these questions may help you. Sara recalled an incident when she had been feeling especially anxious over a problem with a friend. She found herself standing in front of the refrigerator eating one food after another. When she asked herself how she was feeling while she ate, Sara was aware of still feeling the anxiety but somehow of its also being dulled. It seemed to her as if the food were dulling the anxiety, but since food is not a drug she realized that she must have been doing something to herself to alleviate the anxious feelings. After much thought, Sara could see that concentrating on the eating was a *distraction* from concentrating on the incident which had upset her.

Distraction also played a part in Marcia's eating. She realized that during and after a binge, she was so caught up in hating herself for eating that she forgot what was really bothering her. Sometimes it is easier to deal with familiar feelings of self-hate and frustration brought on by overeating than with other more unfamiliar or upsetting feelings. In particular, Marcia had difficulty in letting herself experience anger. It was easier for her to deal with the self-hate associated with her binges than to deal with the angry feelings. Whenever any such feelings began to enter her consciousness she would eat, thereby allowing her to refocus attention on how horrible she felt about overeating and being fat.

Very often I will hear women say they are aware of eating to "push down anger"—as if the food could keep those angry feelings from surfacing and being expressed. In these cases, power is being given to food—the power to push down anger. Yet if the anger is indeed suppressed, it was the woman herself who did the suppressing, attributing it all the while to the food. We will discuss *why* she needs to give the power to the food later on in the chapter.

Let us look at one more example of how my patients have dealt with the question, "What am I doing *to myself* when I put food in my mouth?" Julie was a woman who felt trapped in an unhappy marriage. Her days were boring and repetitive, and there was little joy and pleasure in her life. She realized, after doing the above exercise, that she was turning to food as a source of pleasure. "When I put cake or ice cream or candy in my mouth, I feel good. I get so much pleasure out of the food, it takes my mind off my troubles." Julie was using food to give her what was missing in her life.

This next fantasy will help you discover more specifically what you have given food the power to do in your own life.

Power of Food Fantasy

This fantasy will help you to discover how you have used food in one particular instance. You may find it necessary to repeat the fantasy many times over the next few weeks using different instances in which you were aware of using food to meet emotional needs. For now, however, choose a recent incident in which you used food to make yourself feel better, to keep your mind off troubles, or to give you something to do. You do not have to know why you were eating. All you need to know is that you were eating compulsively. Pick one food at a time, preferably one with which you have had the most difficulty.

Close your eyes and imagine yourself in that situation in which you were eating compulsively. Be aware of your surroundings. Where are you? Is anyone else in the house? . . . Now, picture clearly the food you were eating. (Pause fifteen seconds.) . . . Be aware of its color . . . texture. . . . Where it is placed. . . . Make the picture in your mind as vivid as possible. (Pause twenty seconds.) . . . If the food had a mouth and could talk, what would it want to say to you? (Pause thirty seconds.)

Now, I realize this may be difficult, but I would like you to imagine that you *are* the food—imagine yourself as this food. (Pause twenty seconds.) . . . What is your existence like as the food? (Pause twenty seconds.) . . . What does it feel like to be this food? (Pause fifteen seconds.) . . . Now, as the food, look over at that person who is about to eat you (Pause fifteen seconds.) . . . How does she feel about you? (Pause thirty seconds.) . . . What is she wanting from you? . . . What is she using you for? (Pause thirty seconds.) . . . Can you give that to her? . . . Tell her how you feel (Pause thirty seconds.) . . . Talk some more, letting her respond to what you say (Pause one minute.) . . . Tell her how she could go about meeting her needs without having to eat you. (Pause one minute.)

Now, become yourself again. (Pause fifteen seconds.) . . . Look at the food. Does it look any different to you now? . . . Do you have any greater understanding of how you have used it? (Pause thirty seconds.)

If you wish, you may picture yourself eating the food now. How does it feel? (Pause twenty seconds.)

When you feel ready, open your eyes and come back to your normal existence.

Discussion of Power of Food Fantasy

Though it may seem a little strange at first to imagine yourself as a food, you can gain much awareness from doing the fantasy. This fantasy is most helpful at times when you just do not know why you were eating compulsively. Some women have even been able to stop a binge in progress long enough to try out the fantasy and have then had success in stopping the binge.

Some women realize for the first time, on a gut level, that they have indeed endowed food with magical qualities. Julie saw herself as an ice cream sundae, waiting to be devoured and add more fat to Julie's body. She realized she was using the sundae to put more of a cover over her, as though the extra fat would somehow protect her. Another woman, Suzanna, discovered that her nightly raids on the refrigerator were an attempt to derive enough strength from food to deal with her husband: "No food in the world, though, will give me the kind of strength I need," she finally realized.

Sometimes, your subconscious will get its message across humorously. I often recall the fantasy of one woman, Carol, who had been binging on Ritz crackers for several weeks. During the fantasy, she imagined herself as the personification of a Ritz cracker who proceeded to give her a list of things she was expecting it to do for her. When Carol became herself again and looked at the cracker, it was standing, hands on its "hips," saying indignantly, "You expect me to do *all that?*"

Gaining an awareness of what powers you have given to food is but one step in the process of learning to take care of yourself without relying primarily on food to meet your emotional needs. Just as there was a process of taking the power back from fat, there is such a process involved in taking the power back from food.

Let us go back over the guidelines on p. 29, substituting food for fat, and then I will supply you with an example of how this process unfolds. The process consists of:

1. Uncovering and identifying the functions food has been serving for you both in the past and the present. In other words, "What things have I given food the power to do for me?"
2. Determining *why* you have chosen to use food to meet your needs. "Why did I give the power to food in the first place?" This step may also involve an examination of past as well as present experiences.
3. Exploring why you might not *want* to take the power back from the food.
4. Realizing that food is not doing anything for you. Food cannot pep you up, calm you down, or meet any emotional needs. It is you who are "doing" the things you have attributed to the food.
5. Discovering what exactly you have been doing to calm yourself or energize yourself or forget your troubles, and finding new and perhaps more effective ways than food of meeting your needs.

Let us return to our hypothetical patient, Jenny, whose case we used to illustrate the process of taking the power back from the fat.

In addition to discovering how her fat is functioning in her life, Jenny has been working at uncovering the power she has given to *food* to meet emotional needs. She realizes one day, after the guided fantasy, that she has been giving food the power to "keep angry feelings down . . . I feel like I stuff them down with the food."

As we learned in the chapter on fat, knowing the powers with which the food has been endowed is but a first step. Next, Jenny must explore why she chose to give the power to food to help her deal with anger in the first place. Not surprisingly, Jenny has a lot of difficulty both in allowing herself to feel and to express angry feelings toward others. Her problem is not an uncommon one, since women in our culture have been discouraged from feeling anger, and have very few role models to teach them how the anger can be expressed appropriately. Little girls are often taught to be demure and accepting and above all not to hurt another's feelings. Jenny can remember incidents in which she expressed anger at a parent and was punished, and she recalls angry outbursts at friends for which she was admonished: "Nice girls don't fight." Anger became an unacceptable feeling, to be suppressed and forgotten. Yet anger is a normal emotion, a common result of complex interactions between people, and anger not discharged builds up over time, threatening to overcome and overwhelm. So when angry feelings arise, Jenny quickly turns to food to keep them down. She does not trust herself to keep those volatile emotions under control and so has to give the control to some outside force, in this case, food.

But why did Jenny choose to give the power to *food* to control her feelings? Why not to something else? After all, not all women who have difficulties dealing with anger are compulsive eaters. To find the answer to these questions, Jenny had to go back over her childhood to review her history with respect to food: her earliest food recollections, how food was viewed in her home, who else may have been using food to meet emotional needs. It was at that point that Jenny realized that her mother, who had always been dieting, was like Jenny a compulsive eater. Jenny could remember times her mother would bake cookies "for the kids" and then eat them all herself. Jenny even recalled incidents in which her mother invited her to go out for ice cream after an argument with her husband. Apparently, Jenny's mother had served as a model of how to use food to meet emotional needs. She had actually been taught — albeit unintentionally — to use food this way.

There are many other reasons a woman may have turned to food. A common one is rebellion, using food to disturb someone you wish to displease. Others have learned to use food because food was the only pleasure they were allowed or could afford.

Once you have dealt with why you have given the power to the food, you are ready to explore the third step—why you might not *want* to take the power back. "Of course I want to take the power back," Jenny says. "Now that I know what I'm doing and why, what's to keep me from changing?" Actually there may be much to keep Jenny from changing, and it is important that she face up to these potential obstacles. For instance, Jenny has always used food to hold down the anger. Despite her new awareness she may still fear that without food, the angry feelings would overwhelm her. She does not trust that she knows how to control anger without a crutch.

Each woman has her own reasons for fearing life without food as a crutch. Often it feels like "If I don't use food I'll *have* to face what's bothering me." For one woman, food was a last resort. "No matter how upset I get, I know that I can always reach for the food and feel better. It always works. It's like my panic button. Were I to take the power back from food, what would happen to me? What if I felt overwhelmed with anxiety one day and I didn't have that panic button? It feels like I might go crazy or have a heart attack." Another woman feared the power and responsibility that went with taking power back from food. "It's frightening to think that I'd have the power to take care of my own needs without depending on anyone or anything else. It feels like quite a lot of responsibility."

A third woman felt it was too much of an effort, too hard to take the power back from the food. "There's too much work involved. It's easier to just eat." Another felt, "The power food has over me is much less frightening than the power I might have over myself." She felt she would use her power to destructive ends.

In actuality, when you take the power back from food, you have not lost anything. You do not have to face up to the thoughts and emotions that you have been covering up with food. You will not go crazy and you are not "all powerful." You have been doing all the things you have credited food with; the power really lies within you right now.

Stuffing food down her throat has not kept Jenny's angry feelings from surfacing. Food cannot do that. Jenny has been doing it all along and attributing the power to the food. She does not trust herself, and even if Jenny wants to begin dealing with her anger, letting the feeling through, she does not know how to express it appropriately.

This brings us to the final step—realizing exactly what she has been doing to herself in suppressing angry feelings, and then claiming ownership of her actions (taking the power back). Jenny has two further options at this point. She can work on discovering new ways of calming herself down and accepting angry feelings without using food, or, if she is ready to tackle the issue of expressing anger in her relationships, Jenny could begin testing out ways of expressing what she is feeling. An assertiveness training class might help. In the first instance, Jenny's work would consist of separating a problem in her life (dealing with anger) from the eating problem, an issue we dealt with in the first part of this book. In the second case, Jenny would choose to resolve the problem itself, which would also tend to lessen the compulsive eating. She could even choose to work both on separating the anger problem from the eating and on resolving her difficulties in expressing anger. In both cases Jenny would be taking the power back from the food. She would be learning to meet her needs without using food—an important step in her journey.

This next exercise will enable you to explore what your life would be like if you no longer used food to meet emotional needs.

A World without Food

Close your eyes and imagine yourself in a world where there is no food, and no one has to eat or drink to stay alive. There is no concept of food. Envision yourself going through the day. . . . See yourself waking up in the morning. . . . What do you do when you wake up. . . . How do you start the day? (Pause thirty seconds.) . . . Imagine yourself going through the morning and afternoon. . . . How do you make breaks in the day. . . . How do you rest? (Pause thirty seconds.) . . . What do you do in the late afternoon? (Pause twenty seconds.) . . . What are your evenings like? (Pause twenty seconds.) . . . How do you relate to the other members of your family? (Pause thirty seconds.) . . . What happens when you are upset or a problem arises? How do you deal with it? . . . (Pause thirty seconds.) . . . How do you relate socially with others? (Pause thirty seconds.) . . . How do you celebrate? (Pause twenty seconds.) . . . Spend a few minutes more checking out what it would be like to live in a world without food.

Discussion of A World without Food

Food and eating loom large in our lives. Even those without compulsive eating problems are surprised at the knowledge gained in this fantasy. It is only through imagining your life *without* food that its overwhelming importance to you can be made clear. Our lives, especially as compulsive eaters, revolve around food and eating.

Though the realization of how important food has been in your life is an aim of this fantasy, there is another equally important aim: It can help prepare you for a life without food as a constant source of emotional nourishment, can help you explore ways in which you can cope and function well without using food. Though food has a place of great importance in your life now, it does not always have to be that way.

In analyzing your experience with this fantasy the following questions might help:

1. What did it feel like getting up in the morning?
    If you are accustomed to eating immediately upon arising, as many compulsive eaters (and dieters) are wont to do, you might have felt uncomfortable. If eating were not part of your morning ritual, how else could you start the day? If you are not hungry, must you eat?[2]
2. Did you realize how you use food to mark the transition between one activity and another, or between one part of your life and another?
    In *Fat is a Feminist Issue* Susie Orbach talks of transition eating, which, like punctuation, marks the end of one activity and begins another: for instance, eating after you have completed a chore, before you go onto the next, or the common occurrence of eating as soon as you come into the house. Some of my patients go straight to the kitchen when they come home from

school or work, or from any activity. This eating eases the transition between the outside world and home. For many women who work outside the home, the transition eating allows them time to shift roles from working woman to wife and mother. If you discovered evidence of this kind of eating in your fantasy, can you think of other ways to punctuate your day or ease the transitions other than through food? For example, if you eat every day after work, before you begin making dinner or helping the kids with their homework, can you find new ways to unwind, to create distance between yourself and others to allow yourself time to ease into the new roles? Some women have found taking a shower or bath after work serves the same function that eating had in the past. Others come home and lie down for fifteen minutes or a half hour, with strict instructions not to be disturbed. Still others find that sitting down with a cold drink or a cup of coffee is what they need to relax.

3. What did you learn about how you relate to others through food?

Our society, like most, is food-oriented. Families get together to eat, dinner being the only time some families get together. We meet friends for lunch and socialize over dinner. Even business meetings are often conducted over a meal. Are there other ways to relate to friends and family? If you are not hungry for dinner but desire the companionship of your family, is it necessary to eat? Can you just sit and enjoy being with those you love? For some, family dinner is far from enjoyable. It is an enforced gathering, fraught with tension and fighting. In such cases, eating may be a way of distancing oneself, changing the focus of attention from what is going on around you to the act of eating. If it is not possible to change the way your family relates to one another at dinner, is it possible to find new ways of tuning out?

I recommend trying the fantasy several times — each time checking out in what ways you have been organizing your life around food, perhaps unnecessarily.

Sometimes I suggest to my patients that, when they feel they must get something to eat though they are not hungry, they ask themselves, "What if there were no food in the world and I couldn't eat right now?" At first the concept invokes panic in some, as the following interchange illustrates. This conversation took place between me and a patient over the telephone. The patient, Beth, called one evening because she was in conflict over whether to eat.

> Marion: Beth, you say you want to eat something, because you are anxious. You don't know what's bothering you, but you just have to eat.
> Beth: That's right.
> Marion: Now, I'd like you to imagine something. What would happen if there were no food in the world and you couldn't eat now?
> Beth: (Silence for about fifteen seconds.) I think I would go crazy.
> Marion: *Then* what would happen?
> Beth: I guess I'd have to relax after a while — lie down and try to calm myself down.
> Marion: Do you think you would go a whole day experiencing unbearable anxiety?
> Beth: No, I'd do something to alleviate it. I always do, though it's usually with food.
> Marion: So what makes you feel if you don't face unbearable anxiety *now*, that without food you'll have to face it any more than you already do?
> Beth: I guess I wouldn't. I guess I'd find some other way. It's just that I've never experienced facing life without food.

Perhaps some of your fear of taking the power back from food lies in your lack of experience in facing life without food to help you. This fantasy will help you prepare for such a new life.

Very often women discover that they have been using food to nurture or mother themselves, because they have not learned to ask for what they need from others. Food becomes their main source of nurturance; eating their sole way of self-mothering. The following exercise, which appeared in *Mind Trips to Help you Lose Weight*, will help point out the problem.[3]

Your Own Best Friend

Picture your best friend. Notice the qualities that make this person a best friend. Imagine a situation when you were with this best friend. Picture the way you treat this person. What do you say? What do you do for this person? How do you speak to him or her? How do you deal with this special friend's needs and wants? How do you settle disagreements that come up with the friend?

Now, ask yourself, "Do I treat myself the same way?" Repeat the imagining of how you treat a best friend. Except this time, see yourself as the recipient. Imagine doing all the things for yourself that you would do for a best friend.

Discussion of Your Own Best Friend

Were you surprised to see how poorly you treat yourself compared to how you respond to others' needs? Why should we treat ourselves with less consideration and care and respect than we give to others? It is exactly this lack of self-nurturing and caring which leads to compulsive eating. Food is the only outlet for comfort many women allow themselves. As I have said, we have been neither trained nor encouraged to nurture ourselves. Perhaps it is time we learned. Part of your own inner journey will consist in learning to identify and meet your emotional needs without the use of food. This is learning to nurture and care for yourself. Keep in mind, however, that caring and nurturing yourself does not exclude dependence on others. On the contrary, knowing how to meet your own needs implies knowing when you need to turn to others as well as how to ask for help.

One of the most liberating, though one of the most difficult, aspects of taking the power back from the food is learning to sit with uncomfortable feelings. In our society much emphasis has been placed on ridding oneself immediately of pain or uncomfortable feelings. If you have a headache, take an aspirin; a stomach ache, an antacid; a heartache, go out and find a new lover. So much time and effort is spent avoiding the uncomfortable. Yet, sometimes no amount of drugs or activity or food is going to make you feel better. And *it is okay to feel bad*. It is a natural part of life. Sometimes you may feel sad or anxious or frustrated and you may not be able to do anything about it—*you may not even know why you feel bad*. Often, my patients, upon hearing this permission to feel bad, express great relief: "You mean I don't always have to try and figure things out and I don't have to feel good all the time?" Such an acceptance of the ups and downs of life makes it less likely that a person will turn to food to make things "all better" whenever something goes wrong.

It may be extremely difficult, especially at first, to live with uncomfortable feelings. In fact, it is often necessary to find ways of easing the discomfort. Of course, for the compulsive eater, food has always been the primary means of doing this. As you begin to take the power back from food, you will begin finding new ways of easing discomfort. In my case, I found that as I began to use food less and less to meet emotional needs, new, more effective and acceptable ways of dealing with problems evolved. I use the term "evolve" because that is exactly how the changes came about: I did not set out to look for new ways to deal with problems in my life. For example, as my dependence on food lessened, I found myself doing things I had never done before. I began reading science fiction stories, for example, sometimes reading story after story without stopping to think. Reading science fiction served the same function that eating compulsively had in the past. The stories put me in another world and allowed me to refocus attention from my inner turmoil, creating the needed distance between myself and my problems. Binges had accomplished the same end, but science fiction was much more pleasant. It was always after the fact that I would realize what I had done. Suddenly, the thought would occur to me: "Last night I was upset, and I didn't eat. I didn't even *think* of eating. All I wanted to do was read." Interests in nutrition, running, gardening, and science followed.

My patients are forever looking for their own "science fiction," their own way of dealing with emotional pain without eating, but as long as they emphasize the "without eating," they tend to have little success. The harder one tries "not to eat," the harder the task becomes. I did not arrive at my "science fiction" through will power. As I changed my relationship to food, as I took the power back from food, I began naturally to turn to other ways of dealing with emotional pain—without forethought or planning.

I must warn you, however, of one difficult period through which I, and almost every woman with whom I have worked, had to pass. This step in your journey, which I refer to as the transition period, occurs at the point where food is no longer endowed with great power, but you have not yet developed these other ways of dealing with discomfort and emotional pain. It is an uncomfortable time. You may not know what to do with yourself. You may feel fidgety and anxious but unable or unwilling to eat. I remember even getting angry at my therapists for having brought me to the point where food would not work any more, but nothing else would either (as though it were *their* fault). Yet it is important to keep in mind that this period is only temporary; you will not feel anxious forever. Out of this anxiety will come new, more effective ways of dealing with emotional needs.

Often my patients will ask what to do to stop a binge in progress. I tell them that once you have reached the point of eating in response to some inner discomfort, it is usually too late to stop. You have already made your choice. You are already doing the only thing you think will help. The work has to be done *now*, when you are not binging. You need to explore all aspects of how you have given power to food and why you might fear taking that power back. If you merely try not to eat when you are upset, your efforts will backfire. You will think about eating more. On the other hand, if you work hard at exploring and changing the way you use food, you will begin to change—and it is only *after* you have changed that you will notice what has happened. For instance, you may say to yourself: "I had a fight with my husband last night, and I didn't eat afterward. I didn't even think of eating," or you might realize, as one of my patients did, "I ate some ice cream last night and didn't go back for a second portion. It's not that I exerted my will power. I just forgot to eat any more. That's never happened to me before." It is not that will power is exerted and you resist eating, and it is usually only after the fact that the change in the way you use food becomes apparent.

Before we end our exploration of the "power of food," I would like to return to a point that was touched on earlier in this chapter, a point which is crucial to the understanding of how you have used food in your life. That is that your *beliefs* about yourself and about food are an unbelievably potent force. If you believe food helps you deal with emotional pain, if you believe that food calms you down, peps you up, keeps down anger, makes you happy, *then it does*. On the other hand, if you truly believe and trust that you can take care of yourself, that you can calm yourself down, pep yourself up, without food, then you will do it. You will live up to your expectations of yourself.

If someone you trust gave you a pill to relax you, chances are you would feel more relaxed after taking the pill, no matter what the actual contents of that pill might be. The pill would do what you believed it would do. The same is true for food. That candy you pop in your mouth when you are tense "works" because you believe it will work. You have given it the power to work. "I know that food is not really relaxing me, at least I know it intellectually," you may say, "but I just can't seem to give up that belief. What do I do?" My answer is to refer you back to step 3 in the process of taking the power back from food, discussed earlier in this chapter: Why might you not want to take the power back from the food? You need to explore what it is that is keeping you from facing up to the fact that food has no power to relax you, or do any of the things you have come to expect it to do. Why might you not want to change your beliefs about food?

Once you have found answers to the questions posed in this chapter and have begun taking the power back from food, you will have come a long way in your journey. You will have changed your whole relationship to food. Food will have become just food to you, no longer the "magic" all-purpose drug. You will naturally begin cutting down on your food intake as you turn to food less and less to meet emotional needs. You now are ready to go on to the next step in your journey, a step which extends the body awareness developed in earlier chapters to the area of food.

seven

Putting It All Together and Losing Weight

By now you are well along on your inner journey to giving up your weight problem. You have worked on the powers that you have given to fat and to food to meet emotional needs, and on your fears and expectations about life as a thin woman. You have learned more about your body and explored your body image, and you discovered a new way to eat without resorting to diets. You have no doubt been noticing changes in your eating behavior. Perhaps you no longer binge, or are not as focused on food and diets and fat as you have been in the past. Now, how do you put this new awareness, these changes to work into losing weight and into getting over your eating problem completely?

The work of this final chapter will help you to synthesize your growing awareness and new attitudes into a new approach to your weight problem and to your life. For most of you, this will mean weight loss as well, though for reasons we will discuss, you may have to readjust your concept of how thin you want to get. We will also explore your feelings about giving up your eating problem. Despite the pain and suffering this problem has caused you, there may be some degree of reluctance, some fears about giving it up.

Let us turn our attention first to the matter of losing weight. How thin do you want to be? I am sure there is a number on the scale you envision in your mind. Hard though it may be, I am going to ask you to throw out that vision and rethink your concept of the "right" or "perfect" weight for you. My aim is to help you find the weight at which you feel most comfortable psychologically and physically, and that weight has nothing to do with scales or diet charts. It is a matter of finding the best weight for *you*. How you discover what exactly is the best body weight for you is the focus of this first part of the chapter.

Some of the ideas I am going to present will surprise many of you. I am going to tell you that not everyone was meant to be or can be thin, that some of you may need to readjust your concept of how thin you are going to or "ought" to be. The discussions of diet and weight loss in this chapter are based on the latest research, and they are included not to discourage you, but to help you understand difficulties you may have encountered in losing weight and to help many of you find a more realistic, physically and psychologically comfortable goal for weight loss.

Most of you have been trying constantly to lose weight. Perhaps you have been unable to lose any weight at all, and your weight has been steadily climbing over the years. In short, almost everyone who loses gains back what was lost within a short period of time. Why is this so? In many cases, the reasons for the regained weight are psychological, as we have seen. You might have certain fears about living in your new thin body or expectations for yourself that you did not have as a fat person. You may still need your fat to perform certain functions or meet certain needs. This need for food and fat may have kept some of you from getting thin at all. Yet, in addition to these psychological motivations to gain back or not even give up the weight, evidence is mounting that there are physical abnormalities which contribute to the problem as well. Let us review these findings and explore their implications for those of you with various eating disorders.

Most of this research has been focused on the chemical and hormonal abnormalities that underlie obesity. The results of new studies are appearing at a phenomenal rate, though much of the research is preliminary and the results are not yet conclusive. What emerges from this research is that there are complex physiological processes involved in obesity, and just putting an obese individual on a 1200-calorie-a-day diet regimen will not produce lasting results.

The following discussion of recent research findings will be useful to those of you who are obese. The research being done has helped to debunk some of the myths about overweight people. It is generally believed by the public that fat people eat too much and that it is their gluttonous appetites which are responsible for their extreme obesity. Yet studies indicate this is just not so. Most obese people eat no more than "normal" weight individuals. Many even eat less. While it is not yet clear whether there are physical abnormalties which cause a person to gain weight in the first place, it is now known that once an individual becomes obese, several physical abnormalities may be present which make weight loss more difficult.

According to Judith Rodin, a psychologist at Yale who deals with eating disorders, it may be that some overweight people were overeating during the period when they gained weight, but there is little support for the view that they must continue to overeat in order to maintain their obesity.[1] One explanation for this phenomenon, she continues, is that fat is metabolically more inert than lean. In other words, lean muscle tissue burns up calories at a faster rate than fat. In addition, it has been demonstrated that overweight individuals expend less energy performing activities than their thin counterparts. Other evidence points to an enzyme abnormality discovered in the blood of some obese individuals. In a study done at Boston's Beth Israel Hospital, researchers measured levels of an enzyme ATPase in many obese men and women and found in nearly all cases that blood levels of this enzyme were at least 20 percent below normal. ATPase functions in the body like a pump, transporting sodium and potassium in and out of the cells. According to an article which appeared in the *New York Times*, it has been estimated that "between 1/5 and 1/2 of the body's energy-consuming heat production is caused by the activity of this chemical pumping system."[2] The low levels found in obese individuals suggest that more calories from food are stored as fat, rather than burned for energy. Jeffrey Flier, a physician involved in this research, points out that such a mechanism may have served a useful function in early humans. Since a steady supply of food was not always available, energy had to be conserved efficiently. Reduced levels of ATPase allowed early humans to store food as fat for times of famine. When food was plentiful, ATPase activity would be stepped up, burning up the excess fat stores. Flier postulates that in obese people of our age, that once helpful mechanism is not functioning properly.[3]

ATPase is evidently only one of several mechanisms responsible for regulating weight. Another theory supported by evidence has to do with a substance referred to as "brown fat" which is located around the kidneys, adrenal glands, and between the shoulder blades on the back. This brown fat evidently is responsible for burning up as heat the excess calories a person has consumed. The function of brown fat may help explain why some people can eat as much as they want without gaining weight. All excess food is burned up as heat in individuals who possess greater stores of this tissue. In those who are deficient in brown fat, or in whom the mechanism is defective, weight may be easily gained. Researchers are searching now for drugs which will activate existing brown fat stores in people who are obese.

Other studies have shown that the basal metabolic rate—the amount of energy the body uses while at rest—is lower in overweight people. It is not yet clear whether the reduced rate is the cause of or due to the obesity, but what is clear is that obese individuals burn about 20 percent less energy than normal people, and therefore require 20 percent less food.[4]

Even for the obese woman who is able to lose weight, complications may make keeping that weight off especially difficult. While we have discussed the psychological motivations to regain weight lost, there are, as well, physical reasons why obese women experience difficulty in maintaining the lowered weights. First of all, even after an obese person reduces to "normal" weight, caloric requirements are still lower than for others of the same weight who have never been fat. No one yet knows if this lower need for calories is inherited and a cause of the obesity or the *result* of the obesity itself.

Then there is the fat cell theory, with which you are undoubtedly acquainted. Years ago, it was shown that overeating in early childhood leads to an excess number of fat cells in the body. While there seemed to be no way of reducing the number of cells, it was believed that those who became obese as adults were immune to the problem of excess fat cells. Recent studies have destroyed this notion, indicating that overeating in adults can lead to an increase both in the size and number of fat cells in the body. Although the size of these cells can be diminished through weight loss, the actual number remains the same.

Another study points to the involvement of an enzyme called lipoprotein lipase (LPL) in repeated weight gain in certain obese individuals who are able to reduce. LPL removes triglycerides (a type of fat) from the blood and stores them in the fat cells. The more excess food the body takes in, the more triglycerides are removed from the blood for storage in the fat. Evidently, even moderately obese people have a higher level of LPL than normal weights. In the study obese individuals were placed on a 600-calorie-a-day diet for two or three months, losing an average of 35 pounds. While on the diets, their LPL levels did decrease, but once they resumed a maintenance diet, changes began to occur. Within one week of resuming diets expected to stabilize their new lower weights, LPL levels had risen even higher than what they had been before the start of dieting. It was as though the body increased the enzyme level, in order to help the fat cells gain back what they had lost. Interestingly, once all the weight had been regained, LPL levels dropped back to what they had been previously.[5]

Undoubtedly, as scientists continue to study obesity and its related abnormalities in body functioning, much more will be discovered about the physical causes for obesity and what can be done about them. Eventually one might be able to take a pill which will increase the activity of the body's existing brown fat reserves or even increase the brown fat stores themselves; or a medication might be developed which would lower the concentration of LPL in the blood. But such easy cures are not now available.

Several implications for the obese can be derived from the current research findings. First, it is important to keep in mind that you are not a self-indulgent, gluttonous pig. You may have overeaten to become fat, and some of you may still be eating huge amounts of food, but there may be real physical reasons why you cannot lose weight or keep off the weight you have lost. It serves no purpose to judge yourself harshly or hate yourself because you are fat. This, however, does not mean you did not have psychological reasons to gain weight in the first place, or that you are not holding onto your fat to meet emotional needs, as well. Yet it is important to realize that for whatever reasons you gained weight originally, be they psychological or physical, once you have become obese it is difficult (not impossible) to lose weight permanently. "Does that mean I can never get thin?" you may be asking, feeling discouraged. For a few of you, for now, yes, but for most of you who are obese, these new findings do not necessarily condemn you to a life of unwanted obesity. I did not present them in order to discourage you, but to help you be less self judging. *It really is harder* for you to lose weight than it is for thinner people, and you do not have to hate yourself for not being able to do so all these years. Nonetheless, you can probably get thin — maybe not as thin as you have always envisioned yourself, but considerably thinner. Even though you may need to eat less than most in order to lose or even maintain that loss, if you learn to eat in tune with your body, eating only when hungry and stopping when full, you will be able to get thinner and stay at that lower weight without stringent dieting or a sense of deprivation.

Now let us move on to an examination of the implications which can be derived from research on women who are only slightly "overweight." Many of you may find yourselves in the position of constantly losing and regaining weight; you find yourself gorging until you have gained back every ounce you had fought so hard to lose. There may be a physical component to this pattern in addition to the emotional factors we have discussed. Let us review the concept of "set points" and see how it might relate to your weight problem. According to the theory, the body tends to keep its fat stores at a certain level. When the fat stores fall below that level, the body attempts to regain what it has lost by increasing the appetite. This point at which the body tends to stay is called its set point and is determined, in part, by the number of fat cells in the body. The aim of the body is to keep its fat level fairly constant. This means that if you lose weight and your fat stores fall below a certain level, your body will react by increasing your appetite, so you will eat more food. How do you know what your set point is? Generally, the weight at which you tend to spend the most time would indicate a set point. Therefore, if you often weigh 130 pounds, for example, and despite all attempts to lose ten pounds, still find yourself back at 130, time and time again, then, like it or not, 130 is your set point. Trying to maintain a ten-pound weight loss would be difficult, since your body would attempt to go back to its most comfortable level. In your mind, or on the weight charts, the ideal weight for you may be 120, but your body has different plans. Researchers have been able to identify some factors which influence the body's set point. Diet pills and nicotine tend to lower the set point, but only while they are taken. As soon as you stop smoking or taking diet pills, the set point returns to normal and weight is usually gained. Exercise is the only safe way that has yet been identified to lower the body's set point permanently.[6]

For those of you who are constantly trying unsuccessfully to drop five to ten pounds, there are two choices. You can increase your activity level through a physical conditioning program (running, swimming, even walking) or you can begin to readjust your concept of what constitutes your "ideal" weight. Perhaps you were just not meant to be as thin as you would like. In a society oriented toward extreme slimness, we lose sight of the fact that there are individual differences in body structures and that not every woman was meant to have narrow hips, long legs and a small bust. Perhaps you have been hating yourself for not being able to stick to a diet, lose ten pounds and keep it off—seeing your inability to do so as a personal failure, a sign of a weak character. Aside from subtle unconscious motivations you may have had to hold onto these ten pounds, there could be powerful physical forces at work as well. Isn't it sad that you may have been hating yourself, been miserable with yourself, judging yourself unworthy just because you have not been able to reach a goal which may not be realistic or even possible for you?

Some research studies have shown that an obsession with being thin can be harmful to a person. The effects of anxiety over being even slightly overweight, in addition to the strain on the body of constant weight loss and gain, can be much more devastating to a woman both psychologically and physically than any excess weight ever could.

Furthermore, despite current societal standards and medical

Putting It All Together and Losing Weight

weight charts, the concept of ideal weight is in the process of being revised. The concept of ideal weight has been derived from insurance company standards, but those standards are by no means based on careful scientific study. Evidently, the height-weight charts in use today grew out of attempts by insurance companies in the early twentieth century to identify high-risk customers. It was discovered that policyholders who were overweight tended to die younger than those of less weight. This phenomenon did not mean that being fat *caused* earlier deaths, but that there was an association between the two. The reason for this association was unimportant to the insurance companies, since their aim was only to eliminate customers at high risk. Despite the fact that no causal connection had been established between overweight and early death, the companies endeavored to get their customers to reduce, and by the 1940s a chart of "ideal weights" was in existence. It seems the ideal weight chart was primarily the work of a Louis I. Dublin, who worked as a biologist for the Metropolitan Life Insurance Company. He based his chart on three faulty premises. First was his belief that an individual *should not* gain weight after twenty-five years of age. Secondly, he divided people into three "frame" sizes, though there is no evidence to support such a division. In fact, there still exists no objective measurement of "frame size." Thirdly, he assumed, incorrectly, that people buying insurance represented a fair sampling of the entire population of the country. It was on the basis of these erroneous assumptions that our current weight charts are derived.[7] The doctor who has been authoritatively admonishing you for being ten pounds overweight has been basing his or her judgments of you on outdated, unscientific beliefs.

In recent years, the results of new studies on weight have been published, the most famous and controversial of which is the Framingham study. This study, begun in the 1940s, has followed about half the population of Framingham, Massachusetts throughout their lives. As each person died, the cause of death was determined. In 1980, the researchers concluded that the death rates for women were highest for the very thinnest as well as the heaviest. An article in *Newsweek* stated that "the new mortality tables also show that fashionably skinny isn't necessarily a blessing. In fact, too little weight can be more dangerous than too much. A woman who is 30 percent underweight now appears to face the same hazards as one who is 55 percent overweight."[8] For men, it was found that life expectancy was worst for the thinnest group, and unless the weight was more than 25 percent above average, weight was not much of a factor in life expectancy at all.

However, the Framingham study has its critics. In a study on mice done at the University of California, it was found that mice who were underfed by 60 percent, even as late as "middle age," lived longer and had fewer spontaneous tumors than "normal" control mice. When asked about the Framingham study, one of the researchers, Roy L. Walford, replied, "I don't disagree with the results but with their interpretation—that it is okay to be slightly obese and that it is bad to be thin."[9] He explained that the extremely thin people in the 1980 study were thin not as a result of low-calorie diets, but because of illness. Another researcher has looked over the data on women from the 1980 study and found that if one eliminates the smokers from the thinnest group, they do not, in fact, have the highest mortality.

Clearly, additional studies need to be undertaken to more accurately determine the effects of weight on health, but meanwhile it is becoming evident that we need to rethink our concept of ideal weight. Accordingly, new weight tables are being devised upping the ideal weight about ten pounds.

Finally, let us turn our attention to research which has implications for those of you who are bulimic or who subsist on constant fad or starvation diets in order to maintain a low weight. Thaddeus S. Danowski of the University of Pittsburgh reports that when calorie intake is even moderately restricted by 500 calories, for instance, the body reacts by reducing its BMR (Basal Metabolic Rate). Therefore, to sustain a weight loss "calorie restriction must be substantial and for some people drastic."[10] Another study by the U.S. Department of Health, Education and Welfare in the 1960s, showed that women who lost weight on 1000-calorie-a-day diets experienced a reduction in the BMR and in the calorie intake required to maintain lowered weights. Follow-up studies indicated that reduced calorie diets must be maintained indefinitely in order to maintain the lower weights.[11] They also suggest that exercise is the only safe method known of increasing the BMR. After strenuous exercise, the metabolic rate increases for several hours, in some cases up to twelve hours.

In my own practice, I have seen many women who, after years of dieting strenuously, have lowered their calorie requirements to the point where they cannot eat more than 900-1000 calories a day — otherwise they gain. This phenomenon is believed to have served a survival function in early humans. In times of famine, those who could lower their metabolic rate in response to reduced food intake would be more likely to survive, and though this mechanism serves no function for those of us in twentieth-century Western culture, its effects persist. Those whose eating patterns alternate from starvation diets or fasts to huge binges are in danger of affecting their metabolism, perhaps permanently. Even if you are bulimic, your total caloric intake each day may be low enough to adversely affect your metabolism.

Many of my patients, especially those who are bulimic, have dieted themselves down to weights they consider acceptable and fashionable, but maintain those low weights by subsisting on very little food, laxatives, diuretics, and vomiting. Sometimes these women become so thin that they lose their menstrual periods — certainly a sign that they have become too lean — yet they still feel the need to maintain the low weights. Though not anorexic, these women also have distorted body images and are ignoring their body's messages that they are indeed too thin.

In presenting these research findings, remember it has not been my intent to discourage you, but instead to help you find more realistic goals for yourself and to reduce the negative judgments of your past failures to get thin permanently. These findings can help you discover a weight which is physically most comfortable for your body. It is also important to find a weight which feels comfortable psychologically. The work you have done has been preparation for finding such a weight. If weight is lost slowly, and careful attention is paid to the changes the body is undergoing then you will be giving yourself time to adjust to the changes. You will not need a scale to monitor your weight loss. You will know when you have reached a weight that feels comfortable. Often the women with whom I have worked lose weight in stages. They may lose a number of pounds and then level off for a few months, making adjustments in their feelings about their bodies and getting in touch with any fears they may experience about giving up more fat. Then they will lose some more weight. It does not matter how long the process takes. The point is that when one becomes thin gradually and with awareness of the physical and psychological effects, then the weight loss is likely to be permanent.

One of the ways my patients have prepared themselves for being thin is by imagining themselves thin in various social situations throughout the day. This exercise can be performed several times a day. Ask yourself, "What would it be like, what would it feel like, to be thin in this situation? How would I feel in a thin body now?" Some women try acting "as if" they were thin. They go through a day acting as though they were already living in a thin body, checking out their reactions, as well as what might be different for them.

If you have difficulty envisioning yourself thin, as many who have always been fat do, try seeing yourself five or ten or twenty pounds thinner than you now are. See if you can compact your body in your mind's eye. The more you can see yourself thin, the more of a reality it will become.

Sometimes, a woman will not be able to lose weight or get over an eating problem completely, because the problem itself is serving a function in her life. As we have seen, the constant focus on food and dieting and weight may give a woman a sense of structure in her life. The endless plans to lose weight on this or that diet provide goals in the lives of many women suffering from eating disorders. If one is always striving to get thin (or in the case of some bulimics, stay thin), then one feels a sense of purpose, of moving toward a desired goal. Of course, such a woman can never allow herself to reach her goal for any length of time, or else she will have nothing left for which to strive.

The following fantasy will help you discover if you are having difficulty giving up your eating problem, because the problem itself is serving a function in your life. It will also give you some insights into what functions it is serving and what you can do about it. The fantasy is a variation of one we've already encountered—the personification of the part of you that won't let you get thin (see Chapter 3, "The Reality of Thin").

The Personification of the Part of You That Is Holding Onto Your Eating Problem

Close your eyes and imagine yourself in a meadow at the edge of a forest. . . . It is a bright, sunny day. . . . Above you see the clear blue sky with little puffy white clouds. . . . Out in the meadow you can see wild flowers of many colors and shapes, with butterflies flitting from one to another . . . every now and then you feel a gentle breeze on your face. . . . Spend a while relaxing and enjoying yourself in the meadow. (Pause one minute.)

Now, look toward the forest, and you will notice a path leading deep into the woods. . . . Far away at the end of the path, a figure is coming toward you. . . . You cannot see her clearly yet, but you know that she is the personification of the part of you that will not let you give up your eating problem. (Pause fifteen seconds.) . . . As she approaches you begin to see her more clearly . . . her face . . . her hair . . . her eyes . . . her body . . . the clothes she wears. . . . As she approaches you, she tells you that she is a messenger from your subconscious, and that she is here to tell you why you hold onto your eating problem, why you will not let go of it. . . . Walk with her a bit at the edge of the forest (Pause twenty seconds.) . . . Find a comfortable spot under a tree, and sit down (Pause twenty seconds.) . . . Now she is going to tell you why you are holding onto your problem, how it is functioning in your life. Take a few minutes to listen and then you can ask her questions about what she said. (Pause three minutes.) Ask her what you need to do to begin working on giving up your problem forever. (Pause three minutes.)

Prepare to say goodbye to her for now. (Pause twenty seconds.) . . . She gets up and begins to walk back down the path, then she turns back to you and hands you a gift . . . something which will help you to give up your eating problem. (Pause twenty seconds.) . . . Look at what she gave you. See if you can discover the significance of this gift. (Pause thirty seconds.) . . . She continues back down the path, and you walk back into the meadow. . . . Lie down and relax and give yourself some time to absorb the experience you have just had. . . . (Pause thirty seconds.) . . . And whenever you feel ready, come back to your existence here in the room, and open your eyes.

Discussion of Personification
Some women discover that their eating problem has become so much a part of their identity that it is difficult, often impossible to imagine a life without the problem. One woman, Cheryl, was surprised to hear herself say in the fantasy, "I'd be half a person without the problem. If I didn't have this problem, I wouldn't be me." "Who would I be?" she asked. "I don't know what a Cheryl who didn't have troubles with food and eating would be like. What would she talk about? How would she feel? How would she deal with stress, joy, sadness, guilt, if not with food?" In fact, not only was Cheryl's eating problem a source of identity, but she also discovered that her weight problem makes her different and distinctive. Surrounded by thin women in her upper-middle-class community, she was asserting her differentness by being fat. She could not blend in. But she was also creating an identity with this problem. Everyone knew about it, knew the ups and downs of her diet history as she discussed her problem with all her friends, and so she came to be known in their minds as "Cheryl with a weight problem." It made her distinctive and provided an identity. "Who will I be in relation to others, if I no longer have an eating problem? What will my identity be?" she asked. Especially in those whose eating problems are longstanding, in some cases dating back to infancy, it may be frightening and disorienting to imagine oneself without any eating problem at all. "What would take its place?" one woman asked. "What would I do all day? What would I think about, if I weren't thinking about weight and food and diets?" Another woman experienced a feeling of the floor being pulled out from beneath her and felt herself falling into a deep, black chasm when she tried to picture her life without an eating problem. "My concentration on eating and diets and my body gives me a focus— an orientation—in the world. How would I organize my life without it?" As we discussed, especially for bulimics, the focus on food and eating gives a structure to your life, a structure you may be afraid to give up, for fear that you'll be left in a free-floating, structureless world.

For some, the eating problem provides a goal, something to strive for. In Margaret's case, the goal of weight loss was a constant in her life. It gave her purpose, since she was forever striving to lose weight. Yet she was never able to lose all the weight she wanted and did not know why. The personification told her that she could not permanently lose the weight and thus give up the problem, because to do so would be to give up the only goals she had in life. Without the goal of weight loss, she would have to face the reality that she was stagnating, had ceased growing emotionally, professionally, and socially. The intense focus on losing weight was providing her with a false sense of purpose and movement in her life. The personification also told her that in order to give up her eating problem permanently, she would have to take a more critical look at her life, examine why she was stagnating and decide what to do about it. This realization of how she had been using the eating problem to cover up a real sense of lack of fulfillment led Margaret into therapy.

Another woman, Patty, also discovered that her eating problem was serving a function in her life. At times in her life when she felt the need to pull back, to slow down, to escape her unrealistically high expectations for herself, she would gain weight—up to seventy or eighty pounds. Then Patty would withdraw from the world, stay at home and isolate herself from others for some time; when she felt ready to venture out into the world again, she would lose the weight. Each cycle took several years, but there was a definite pattern to her weight loss and gains which corresponded to different needs at different periods of her life. During the time she was in one of my groups she lost eighty pounds. She felt ready to move out into the world, to develop her business, and so was able to give up the weight. She kept the weight off for almost a year, but when she began feeling the need to stay home again, she began to gain back the weight. After several months of weight gain, Patty returned to me, confused and disappointed in herself. Through the personification fantasy she was able to uncover this pattern of losing and gaining. She learned that when her business began to fail it meant that she would have to go to work for someone else in a nine-to-five job, a prospect which angered and frustrated her. She needed to withdraw from the outside world, to remain safely at home with her children, rather than face the prospect of such a job. The only way Patty would allow herself to do this was by getting fat. If she became fat, she thought she had no choice but to stay home. If she were thin, she thought she had no choice but to look for a new job.

Patty began to see a pattern to her life which followed the one she was presently experiencing.

Once Patty identified this pattern, the first step had been taken in giving it up, but the harder work lay ahead—that of disconnecting her eating problem and weight from the other problems in her life. Patty's work was to first own up to her ambivalence about work and to the fact that at this time, regardless of what she *believed* was the right thing to do, she needed to stay home. She had to be able to envision herself thin, without an eating problem *and* home, not working nine-to-five, in order to give up her eating problem for good. If thin still meant "out there working," then Patty would not allow herself to be thin. She also began to examine her unrealistically high expectations for herself when thin.

Sometimes, it is the obsession with eating, fat, or dieting itself which is serving a function in a woman's life. Linda's personification told her that by obsessing about food she was keeping her other problems at bay. "As long as I am focused on food, I don't have to focus on anything else. I don't have to think about or feel anything else. If I gave up my eating problem, and I no longer obsessed about food, I'd be flooded with feelings and problems. I couldn't face that." Clearly, the obsession has served this woman well, and it would be difficult for her to give up her problem completely until she began to trust that she could take care of herself, that she would not be flooded with emotions were she not so focused on food. Just as others have given power to fat or to food, Linda has given power to her obsesssion to keep unwanted thoughts and feelings at bay. She fears that to let go is to open the floodgate. Yet it is not the obsession but Linda, herself, who has kept these emotions and thoughts under control, and she could do so even without her obsession.

Consider the following questions in analyzing your own fantasy:

1. What form did the personification take? Just as in the fantasy from "The Reality of Thin," the form in which the personification presented itself to you may give some clues as to its meaning.

2. Did you discover that your eating problem was serving a function in your life? If so what are you using it for and how can you begin to find new ways to meet those needs? One woman, Carla, learned from her fantasy that her need for structure and purpose was underlying her inability to give up the eating problem for good. Bored with being a housewife, she had turned to eating as a way of filling in time, structuring her days around meals and providing herself with a sense of purpose in her daily life. She did not want to go to work full-time, but did find the idea of returning to art school part-time an exciting prospect. As she got involved in art school her need for structure and purpose became increasingly fulfilled by her new endeavors. Carla realized that she had come a long way toward giving up her eating problem when she became so engrossed in a painting that she forgot to eat, and realized with astonishment that those sensations she had been feeling in her stomach in the past few hours were pangs of hunger.

In order to give up your eating problem permanently, you too may have to make fundamental changes, finding new ways to orient yourself in the world, to provide yourself with structure or to develop a sense of purpose in your life.

3. What was the significance of the gift your personification gave you? The gift itself has a meaning for you. What was the personification trying to tell you by giving you this particular gift? One woman, Beth, who discovered she feared giving up her eating problem because it was so much a part of her self-identity, was given an empty book by the personification. At first the meaning was unclear, but gradually Beth came to understand that in giving up her eating problem and in getting thin, she was forging a new identity for herself. The personification had given her a new book, ready for her to fill up. The process of finding a new identity could be an exciting one as Beth began to "write" her life anew. Rather than fearing the unknown, Beth began to look forward to creating her new identity without fat or food. Another woman, Cindy, received a clock, with the implied message that she needed to give herself time to change. "My personification was giving me the gift of time, assuring me that I would be able to give up my eating problem,

but helping me to see that this problem had been so much a part of my life for so long that patience and time would be needed before I could let go of it forever."

What was the implied message of your own gift? At first the message may not be apparent, but keep working at it. Eventually the meaning of the gift will become clear to you.

Now we enter the final stages of our journey together. Remember that getting thin and staying there is not an end in itself. There is a tendency to look at "thin" as an end, a point at which you've arrived, but by now you should be beginning to see that being thin is nothing more than being thin. Thin does not mean "together," happy, sexy, outgoing, energetic, or any of the other qualities you and our culture have placed on it. Thinness is merely a state or condition of your body, in which the fat tissue is minimal. Getting thin is not a great accomplishment in the sense that it will not provide you with unending happiness and an end to your troubles in life. If you look at your entire life as a journey, getting thin isn't an end in itself—just a part of the process.

Having put "thinness" in perspective, let us now turn to how one gives up the weight. At this point, all our work will come together into a cohesive whole. By now you have become aware of how fat and food have been functioning in your life and of the powers which you have given them. You have taken much or most of the power back, as you no longer need food and fat to meet emotional needs. You have worked through your fears and unrealistic expectations about life as a thin person and have a fairly realistic picture of what to expect both from yourself and from others when you get thin. You have perhaps readjusted your concept of how thin you are going to be. Your ability to discern and attend to internal body signals has been finely tuned; and basically, you know when you are hungry, when you are full, and what foods will be most satisfying to you. If you have not already begun doing so, you are now ready to lose weight.

For some of you the process of weight loss may have already begun, especially since you are no longer consuming the quantities of food you used in the past to meet emotional needs. Others of you may find that though you no longer binge, no longer consider yourself a compulsive eater, you are eating just enough to maintain your present weight. For those of you in this position, it may be necessary to do some more work on why you may not want to give up your weight or your eating problem. Perhaps there are physical factors, discussed earlier in this chapter, which are preventing you from losing at this point. In that case you will need to fine-tune your ability to eat when you are hungry and stop when you are full to the point that you are eating less, or more likely (and a healthier alternative), you may need to take up some form of physical exercise to increase your metabolism.

"How do most of your patients lose weight?" I am often asked. Usually one of two things occurs. Either the woman loses interest in food for a time, eating only because she needs to—a phenomenon which amazes even those women to whom it is occurring—or the ability to eat only when hungry and stop when full becomes so finely tuned that very little food is eaten. In either case, there is no willful attempt at dieting. There is no sense of deprivation, especially since there are no self-imposed restrictions on what can be consumed. Women have lost weight on ice cream sundaes five times a day, when the amount of ice cream eaten corresponds to the body's internal sense of when it needs to be fed and how much. Two spoonfuls or two cups may suffice at any given time. By presenting this example, I do not mean to imply that you should create a diet for yourself based on ice cream, five times a day. In fact, it is likely that your body would not crave such a diet for long, but I offer this example to show you that when you are eating "in touch" with your body's needs, there is no need to count calories or deny yourself any foods. Your body knows how much food it needs, without external counting and measuring. Just let go and trust, paying careful attention to what your body is telling you, and your body will naturally move toward the body weight at which it most comfortably functions.

Remember, this is not a diet program I propose, but a process of giving up excess weight—a process that comes from inside, not imposed by external authorities and constrictions. And, because it is a process, it unfolds slowly. Do not expect to drop ten pounds a week, as you would on the latest fad diet. You are not on a diet program, but instead are turning inward and allowing a natural body process to unfold. The slow weight loss, independent of outside structure or authority, is more likely to be permanent. For those who are obese, the process may take some time, and weight may be lost in stages, with weeks, perhaps even months between periods of weight loss, during which time your body and mind will have time to adjust to the changes.

Though for most of you weight loss is your goal, your reason for embarking on this journey, to me the aims are somewhat different. I would consider your journey successful if foods and fat are no longer great issues in your life, if you no longer structure your day around food, diets, and daydreams about getting thin, if you no longer hate yourself for having any fat on your body, if you no longer or rarely binge (or vomit). In other words, my goal for you has been to help you get over your eating problem. If you have lost weight, as well, that is good, but I do not consider you a failure if you do not get thin.

You may find after some time that the nonjudgmental, accepting attitude you have learned with respect to your eating problem is beginning to generalize into other areas of your life. You may be becoming less compulsive about many things other than just food and eating. You may become more accepting and loving of yourself in many ways. This inner journey to give up your weight or eating problem is but a beginning. There is so much more to learn. You might even begin to look at your journey of self-discovery as an adventure. I do.

Good Luck.

A Note to Psychotherapists

It is my hope that this book will provide other psychotherapists as well as the general public with specific treatment approaches to compulsive eating disorders. It would take another book to explain fully the underlying concepts of my approach in psychotherapeutic terms, but this short chapter will provide you with some ideas as to how my work can help you in your own practice.

Let me state at the outset that I do not claim to have *the* answer to compulsive eating disorders, nor do I expect you to agree with everything I have said. You can take from what I have presented that which makes sense to you and then apply it in your own way. This chapter merely provides you with clues as to how this material can be used. Before discussing specific treatment techniques, however, there are several general points I want to make about how I view the psychotherapeutic treatment of eating disorders.

First, it is implicit in my approach that eating disorders are multidetermined. One cannot pinpoint a single event or predisposing factor and say "this is the cause of Mrs. Smith's eating problem." Perhaps there was a problem in early infancy in the mother-daughter feeding relationship, but that problem alone would be insufficient to produce an eating disorder. Instead, there were likely several other predisposing factors—genetic, psychological, physiological, and environmental—which interacted and led to the development of the disorder. For instance, you may have a case, Mrs. Smith's, in which you have determined that there were indeed problems in the interplay between mother and child in infancy, especially around feeding behavior, which led to certain difficulties in hunger awareness. In addition, Mrs. Smith's father may have been obese due to certain metabolic disturbances. Mrs. Smith may have inherited these abnormalities as well as her father's large body type. Her mother may have, herself, used food to meet emotional needs. As a teenager, Mrs. Smith may have befriended a group which valued highly thin, stylish bodies, and in her attempt to meet that standard, she may have dieted relentlessly, thus further upsetting her body's metabolism. Still trying desperately, but unable to fit her body into the unrealistically thin image, Mrs. Smith may have begun vomiting some of her daily food intake. The result: a bulimic. The cause: Surely not the disordered mother-child relationship alone. It was the interaction of the early childhood experiences with the genetic and physical factors and the peer group pressures which led to the bulimic behavior. Had Mrs. Smith had a different genetic or metabolic makeup, had her peer group valued "intellectual development" rather than low body weights, she would probably never developed an eating disorder or her eating problems would have been much less severe.

In evaluating a patient, therefore, it is important to keep in mind the multidetermined nature of the disorder. Look for predisposing factors as well as factors which perpetuate the disorder—secondary gains, metabolic and behavioral abnormalities caused by severe chronic caloric restriction or obesity, the addictive nature of vomiting, and so on. Treatment must be based on the individual's unique profile. To treat Mrs. Smith on the basis of her early childhood distortions alone would do her a disservice. Work would also have to be done on the power of food, on eating awareness, and perhaps on accepting the reality of a body which cannot be as thin as she feels it should be. If it is determined that there are no secondary gains from the fat, or that she has not given her fat the power to help her cope in the world, then those areas need not be dealt with in the therapy. The treatment will be based only on the various factors which went into producing and perpetuating the individual's eating disorder.

A Note to Psychotherapists

Eating disorders vary from anorexia to obesity. In fact, one can view the eating disorders on a continuum:

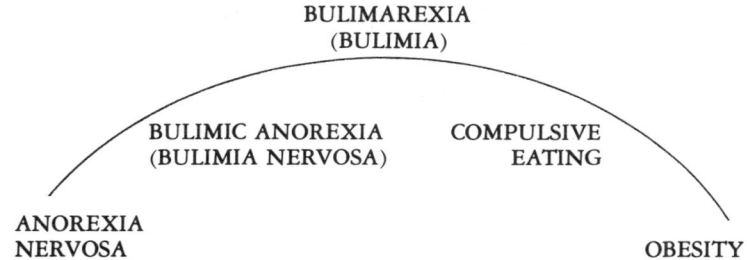

There is much confusion in the profession over the various terms. For the purposes of this book, it is less important exactly where you place a patient on the continuum or the exact term you use to descibe her, as it is to look at those underlying predisposing and perpetuating factors. One would work differently with a bulimic who was anorectic than with the bulimic who throws up once or twice a day because her friends are doing it. The concepts in this book are applicable for the most part to those women who fall in the area from bulimarexia through obesity. (Bulimarexia is defined here as the woman who binges and purges but whose weight falls within ten pounds of normal.)

Psychotherapists have traditionally tended to treat fat and eating as symptomatic of an underlying disorder. Treatment consists of working on the underlying emotional disorder rather than the symptom, with the expectation that the disordered eating behaviors or the weight will disappear once these issues have been resolved. Such is not the case. I have treated many women who have had years of therapy, and while they may have made enormous changes in several areas of their lives, their eating problems remained.

Instead of ignoring the "symptom," the approach I have presented takes the symptom—the fat, the disordered eating—and looks at how it has been functioning in the patient's life. The symptom itself is a focus of treatment. It is explored rather than ignored.

Another way to look at how this approach to eating problems differs from traditional psychotherapeutic approaches was discussed in the chapter "The Power of Fat." One can look at the fat or eating problem as a ball in the center, and radiating out from that ball will be problem areas in a woman's life.

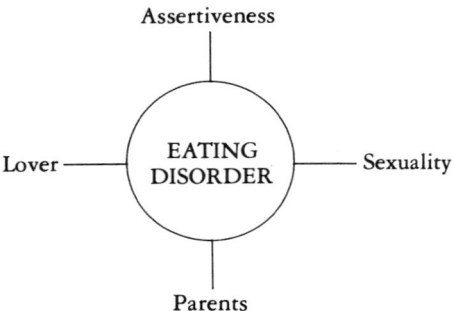

The work of the therapist using my approach is to break the connection between the compulsive eating or fat problem and the other problem areas in a woman's life. Though there is some exploration and discussion about those particular problem areas which have become entangled with the eating disorder, the focus of the psychotherapy is to unhook the eating behavior from them rather than resolve the other problems themselves. In the case of Mrs. Smith, for example, the woman may have problems with assertiveness, especially in expressing anger. She may have sexual difficulties with her lover. Our work in treatment would be to explore how she has associated her body weight and her eating with these problems and how she might break those connections. She would still presumably have difficulties arising from her relationship with her lover. Her sexual problems would not necessarily be resolved and she still might not be able to express anger all the time, but she would no longer be using food and weight to deal with those and other problems in her life. Of course, it is likely that she might have made some progress in dealing with her sexuality or in expressing anger directly instead of through eating, but for the most part the focus would have been not on resolving these issues completely but on separating them from food and body weight. For this very reason, those patients of mine who have been

A Note to Psychotherapists

or are in general therapy are often most successful. The two approaches, coming from opposite ends, tend to complement each other well.

In order to work effectively with women with eating disorders, one must be clear about one's own views of fat and thin. Any judgments will somehow be expressed on some level in the treatment process. Often when teaching or supervising other therapists, I will have them draw up a "fat is . . . thin is . . ." list, like the one which appeared in chapter 2. The purpose of this list is not so much to get at the therapist's unconscious needs for fat, but to uncover beliefs and opinions that will inevitably be conveyed to the patient. For instance, if "out of control," "disgusting," and "gluttonous" were to appear on your "fat is . . ." list, it is likely that your obese patients will perceive your true feelings about fat and that these unconscious judgments will hinder their progress in subtle or not so subtle ways: "If my therapist thinks I'm digusting, then I must be." Similarly, if the therapist thinks being thin is wonderful and will bring a woman happiness, these thoughts will be conveyed to the patient as well, reinforcing her belief that getting thin will be the answer to all her problems.

It is therefore important for any therapist who plans to work or already works with people with eating disorders to become aware of those underlying, sometimes unconscious beliefs and judgments about body weights and eating behaviors. Once the beliefs and judgments are uncovered they can at least be worked on so that they will interfere as little as possible in the psychotherapeutic process.

Some common beliefs that may interfere with treatment include:

1. *Compulsive eating is a sickness.* It is *not* a sickness, but a way in which the individual has learned to cope with other problems in her life. Compulsive eating serves a protective function and your job is to help the patient uncover its protective function and find new ways to meet her needs.
2. *Overeating results from lack of will power.* Compulsive eating serves a function. It is a defense. The compulsive eater uses food and fat to meet certain emotional needs. It is not more will power or motivation which is needed, but an exploration of

how the problem is functioning in the patient's life, and an attempt to find new, more direct, more effective ways of getting what she needs.
3. *Everyone who is fat overeats. Fat people are gluttonous.* As we saw in Chapter 7 it is not clear that all fat people eat more than thin people or that, once fat, a person must continue to overeat to maintain the excess weight.
4. *Everyone can be thin. It's just a matter of will power.* As pointed out in the last chapter, not everyone was meant to be thin. A person's normal set point may be much higher than the norm and no amount of dieting will change the set point — the body will always exert pressure to return to its own "normal" level of fat.
5. *Fat is ugly and disgusting.* It is not fat in itself that is ugly, but our cultural training that influences our perception. In addition, fat women who manage to get past societal standards of beauty, and who feel good about their bodies and themselves no matter what their weight, *are* beautiful.
6. *Fat is unhealthy.* Yes and no. While excess fat has been associated with many physical problems, the causal connection between fat and particular physical disorders is not yet clear. One must look at the individual and determine if that particular person's excess fat is causing or contributing to a health problem. If it is clear that the fat is endangering the person's health and she still holds onto it, she must have some pretty strong motivations to hold onto the food and fat which override her desire for health. Your work would be to uncover those motivations.

As you can see, working with eating disorders may require some cognitive restructuring on your part as well as the part of the patient. It may be necessary to explore your own belief system first so that you can help the patient look at her own.

In fact, much of the work presented in this book can be viewed as a form of cognitive restructuring — of examining beliefs the patient may have about her eating and her weight and helping her to change those beliefs, thereby easing her problem. For example, if the patient believes that she is bad and weak-willed for overeating, these beliefs will have an effect on her eating. Binges have two components.[1] The first consists of eating to meet some emotional need. The second part of the binge results from negative self-judgments about the initial eating behavior: "What's wrong with me? Why can't I control my eating? I'm weak. I'm bad." In response to those judgments, the compulsive eater binges some more. Once the woman has examined and reevaluated her need to eat — once she has begun to view compulsive eating as a protective mechanism which has allowed her to cope with feelings she felt incapable of handling any other way — the second aspect of the binge is eliminated. There are no judgments, no bad feelings about herself for having eaten to avoid anger, so there is no continuation of the binge.[2]

Now that we have covered the overall approach to eating disorders, let us turn to how you, as a psychotherapist, can make use of my book in your own practice. To a large extent, what you take from my book and how you apply it will depend on your psychotherapeutic orientation. Strictly psychoanalytic therapists would not be able to apply directly the material presented here, but the concepts might present them with a new way of thinking about fat and food and the defensive function of eating. They might also consider referring a patient to another therapist for treatment of the specific eating disorder while the general individual therapy continued. (I recognize the objection of many psychoanalytically oriented therapists that such action would promote a split transference, but such has not been the case due to the nature of the eating disorder therapy.) Those therapists who take a more eclectic approach may choose to incorporate the more specific methods of dealing with the eating disorder contained in my book.

There are those who will view the approach I have presented here as basically psychoanalytic, with its emphasis on uncovering unconscious motivations to be fat and to eat, and some will view the work as a form of ego supportive therapy, aimed at strengthening ego functions which relate to cognition, self-esteem, body image, and discerning emotional and physical states. Others dismiss the approach as merely behavioral. The approach I have presented has its roots in many different therapeutic approaches; yet no matter how I am working — be it in strengthening ego functioning, uncovering unconscious associations, changing maladaptive behavior — my focus is on food, body weight, and the eating disorder itself. I am not interested in strengthening ego functions per se, but only as they relate to problems with food. I am not aiming at uncovering just any unconscious material, but only that which relates to the eating disorder.

In my work I take on many roles in addition to that of psychotherapist. My work with eating disorders is more directive and dynamic than it is with other problems. I take on the role of educator — teaching the women how to relax, how to be more assertive, how to listen to the body. I act as a role model as well (especially effective because I myself have overcome an eating problem).

Treatment of eating disorders is, in my experience, most effective when carried out in a group setting, though I work individually as well. The exercises and guided visualizations presented in my book are conducive to exploration within a group, each woman sharing her own experiences with the other group members. The support system which arises in my groups is helpful, especially while the women are struggling to give up old beliefs and behaviors which society has reinforced and continues to reinforce: beliefs such as, "You must diet to lose weight"; "If you eat one cookie you'll eat them all"; "Compulsive eaters are weakwilled"; "Fat people are undeserving." The women draw on each other for support as they struggle against their culture's view of food and fat. Individual treatment will yield results, but generally more slowly. Sometimes I will see a woman both individually and in group, especially when there is a need for treatment more than once a week.

Whether in group or individually, I generally begin the work with the focus on eating awareness, emphasizing nonjudgmental awareness of eating behavior. I will have the patient observe her hunger for a while — its physical sensations, its emotional meanings. Then I will have the woman attempt to wait until she is hungry before she eats. Following the sequence presented in "Eating Awareness," I will teach the woman to listen to body signals. Slowly, even before the eating awareness work is completed, I move into the other aspects of the problem. My role slowly shifts from teacher to therapist as we begin to explore the role

A Note to Psychotherapists

food and body weight are playing in this woman's life. As I work, I keep in mind the framework presented in "The Power of Fat" and "The Power of Food," which shapes the process of taking the power back from food and fat. Once one is aware of what powers the woman has given to food and to her fat, it is necessary to do more exploration, so that she can begin to meet her emotional needs in ways other than through the use of food and body weight. Knowing that she has given food the power to allay anxiety is not enough to effect changes in the eating behavior. One must also explore why power was given to food in the first place, and why this person needed to turn to *food* to calm herself. Where and when did she learn to use food? Why might she not want to take the power to allay anxiety back from food? Such questions give shape and direction to the therapeutic interactions.

Finally, let me touch briefly on the topic of guided visualizations. It is not absolutely necessary to use the guided visualizations in order to put the ideas I have presented in this book into practice. In fact, in some individuals such an approach would be contraindicated. However, in a relatively healthy individual capable of using the visualizations effectively, their use can speed up the process of uncovering unconscious motivations to hold onto fat, fears and expectations about being thin, and emotional needs for food. They can be used both diagnostically and prescriptively. For those patients who cannot work with guided visualizations, other exercises such as the "fat is . . . thin is," list may be of some help in uncovering unconscious material. Sometimes, especially in the case of the guide fantasy, I will make an audio tape for patients who want to work on the visualizations at home. Often they find the tape useful for relaxation purposes even if no new material is uncovered.

I hope I have been able to provide you with a new perspective on eating disorders and some practical ideas as to how they can be treated. There is much to learn in this still-new field. I wish you luck in your own work.

Notes

Introduction

1. The percentage of dieters who regain their weight is believed to be between 90 and 97 percent.
2. In *Directing the Movies of Your Mind* (New York: Harper & Row, 1972), Adelaide Bry makes the point that though a person may consciously want to attain a goal, at an unconscious level he or she may be resisting that goal. She writes, "It's even possible that you know, deep down, that what you believe you need isn't *really* what you need" (p.41). It is my experience that these unconscious conflicts are likely to undermine even the suggestions presented to you during hypnosis.
3. For an in-depth analysis of the relation between fat and woman's position in our society, read *Fat is a Feminist Issue* (New York: Berkley Books, 1979) by Susie Orbach.

Chapter One   My Journey: Bulimia

1. Carlyle C. Douglas, "The Gorging—Purging Syndrome: A New Clue to Overweight," *Moneysworth* (October 1977): 10.
2. Susan Squire, "Why Thousands of Women Don't Know How To Eat Normally Anymore," *Glamour* (October 1981): 309.
3. Ibid., p. 309.
4. Jane Brody, "An Eating Disorder of Binges and Purges Reported Widespread," *New York Times* (October 20, 1981): C1.
5. Ibid., p. C1.

Notes

Chapter Two The Power of Fat

1. For other similar guide fantasies, see Irving Oyle, *The New American Medicine Show* (Santa Cruz, CA: Unity Press, 1979), and the advisor fantasy in Adelaide Bry's, *Directing the Movies of Your Mind*, (New York: Harper & Row, 1972): 78.
2. In my groups I usually accompany the guide fantasy with Steve Halpern's *Spectrum Suite* (Halpern Sound, 1775 Old Country Rd #9, Belmont, CA 94002).

Chapter Three The Reality of Thin

1. The idea for this exercise was given to me by Robin Halpern, a former group member, now a therapist herself.
2. The idea for this exercise was given to me by Nancy Kahn, a friend and colleague.

Chapter Four Bodywork

1. Hilde Bruch, *Eating Disorders* (New York: Basic Books, 1973), p. 89. The statements in parentheses are my additions.
2. Seymour Fisher, *Body Consciousness* (New York: Jason Aronson, 1974), p. 21.
3. Judith Thurman, "Never Too Thin to Feel Fat," *Ms.* (September, 1977).
4. Orbach, *Fat is a Feminist Issue*, p. 89.
5. Fisher, *Body Consciousness*, p. 37.
6. William Bennett and Joel Gurin, "Do Diets Really Work?" *Science '82* (March 1982): 47.
7. Kathryn Lance, *Getting Strong* (New York: Bobbs-Merrill, 1978) p. 212.

Chapter Five Eating Awareness

1. For a further discussion of the problems inherent in dieting, read the chapter on hunger in Orbach, *Fat is a Feminist Issue*, and William Bennett and Joel Gurin, *The Dieter's Dilemma* (New York: Basic Books, 1982).
2. Bruch, *Eating Disorders*, p. 45.
3. Timothy Gallwey, *The Inner Game of Tennis* (New York: Random House, 1974), p. 45.
4. Orbach, *Fat is a Feminist Issue*, pp. 109-10.
5. Leonard Pearson and Lillian Pearson, *The Psychologist's Eat-Anything Diet*, (New York: Wyden, 1973), pp. 32-33.
6. Don Gerrard, *One Bowl* (New York: Random House, 1974) p. 19.
7. Ibid, p. 26.
8. Ibid, p. 26-27.

Chapter Six The Power of Food

1. It is true that there is some evidence that food can affect your thoughts and feelings to some extent, especially in the case of those who are sensitive to a particular food (see, "In Pursuit of Love: Three Current Studies" *The New York Times* (January 22, 1980): C2); yet what I am referring to is the sense of feeling better as soon as the food enters the mouth, long before it has been metabolized and could affect one physically.
2. For those of you who are hypoglycemic or have other medical problems, it may be necessary for you to eat soon after rising whether you are hungry or not.
3. Frances Meritt Stern and Ruth S. Hoch, with Jean Carper, *Mind Trips to Help you Lose Weight*, (New York: Playboy Press, 1976) p. 164.

Chapter Seven Putting It All Together and Losing Weight

1. John Langone, "Girth of a Nation," *Discover* (February, 1981): 58.
2. Harold Schmeck, "Research into Body's Chemistry May be the Key," *The New York Times* (February 24, 1981): C2.
3. "Why You Can't Lose Weight," *Newsweek* (December 8, 1979): 109.
4. "Girth of a Nation," p. 58.
5. "Research into Body's Chemistry May Be Key," p. C2.
6. William Bennet, and Joel Gurin, "Do Diets Really Work?" *Science '82* Vo. 3(2) March 1982, p. 47.
7. Ibid, p. 49.
8. "Why You Can't Lose Weight," p. 109.
9. "Belt-Tightening for a Longer Life," *Science News* (March 6, 1982): 152.
10. Dava Sobel, "Nutritional Factors: What Does Dieting Really Do?" *The New York Times* (February 24, 1981): 2.
11. U.S. Department of Health, Education and Welfare, *Obesity and Health* (1966) p. 60. Washington, D.C.

A Note to Psychotherapists

1. I owe my understanding of the two-part nature of binges to Sandra Haber, New York City.
2. For a detailed discussion of the conceptual disturbances in anorexia, see David Garner and Paul Garfinkel, *Anorexia Nervosa: A Multidimensional Perspective* (New York: Brunner Mazel, 1982). It is my experience that these disturbances characterize women with other eating disorders as well. The Garner and Garfinkel book is also an excellent examination of the multidimensional approach to the treatment of anorexia. I highly recommend it.

Suggested Readings

Beller, Anne Scott, *Fat and Thin: A Natural History of Obesity* (New York: Farrar, Straus & Giroux, 1977).
Bennett, William and Joel Gurin, *The Dieter's Dilemma* (New York: Basic Books, 1982).
Bry, Adelaide, *Directing the Movies of Your Mind* (New York: Harper & Row, 1972).
Chernin, Kim, *The Obsession* (New York: Harper & Row, 1981).
Gallwey, Timothy, *The Inner Game of Tennis* (New York: Random House, 1974).
Gendlin, Eugene, *Focusing* (New York: Everest House, 1978).
Gerrard, Don, *One Bowl* (New York: Random House, 1974).
Kaplan, Jane Rachel, *A Woman's Conflict: The Special Relationship Between Women and Food* (Englewood Cliffs, New Jersey: Prentice Hall, 1980).
Lance, Kathryn, *Getting Strong* (New York: Bobbs-Merrill, 1978).
LeShan, Eda, *Winning the Losing Battle* (New York: Bantam, 1981).
Millman, Marcia, *Such a Pretty Face: Being Fat in America* (New York: W.W. Norton, 1980).
Orbach, Susie, *Fat is a Feminist Issue* (New York: Berkley Books, 1979).
Orbach, Susie, *Fat is a Feminist Issue II* (New York: Berkley Books, 1982).
Pearson, Leonard and Lillian, *The Psychologist's Eat Anything Diet* (New York: Wyden Books, 1973).
Vincent, L.M., *Competing with the Sylph: Dancers and the Pursuit of the Ideal Body Form* (Kansas City: Andrews & McMeel, 1979).

For the Mental Health Professional:

Boskind-Lodahl, Marlene, "Cinderella's step-sisters: A feminist perspective on anorexia and bulimia," *Signs: Journal of Women in Culture and Society.*

Bruch, Hilde, *Eating Disorders: Obesity, Anorexia and the Person Within* (New York: Basic Books, 1973).

Garner, David and Garfinkel, Paul, *Anorexia Nervosa: A Multidimensional Perspective* (New York: Brunner/Mazel, 1982).

International Journal of Eating Disorders Van Nostrand Reinhold (135 West 58th Street, New York, New York 10020).

Index

ANAD (Anorexia Nervosa and Associated Disorders), 18
Anorexia, 12
Assertiveness training, 16, 33, 67, 86, 152
ATPase, 162-63

Beth Israel Hospital (Boston), 162
Bingeing, 18-24, 25, 136
   control, need to feel in, 22-24, 25
   food denial and, 74, 113
   purposes of, 18-24
      being good to oneself, 22
      case examples, 18-24
      defense against anxiety and depression, 22
      escaping high expectations, 21-22
      expression of anger, 19-21
   stopping binge in progress, 158
Binge-purge syndrome, 7-8, 12, 14
BMR (Basal Metabolic Rate), 168-69
Body, awareness of, 81-110
   "accepting the fat," 83-84, 88-91, 102-03
   aluminum foil figure exercise, 102
   drawing of self exercise, 96-101
   "Expansion of self" fantasy, 95-96
   importance of, 89-90
   merging of physical and psychological body boundaries, 91-92
   mirror exercises, 92-95
   tracing outline of self exercise, 101-02
   body image defined, 81-82
   differing concepts of body, 82-83
   emotions and, 85-86
   misinterpreted sensations taken for hunger, 86, 107, 113
   negative and distorted images, 83-84, 86-88
   distrust of body, 84-85
   fear of body, 85
   See also Clothing, significance of; Exercise (physical)

Body Consciousness, 91, 107
Boskind-Lohahl, Marlene, 13
Brown fat, 163, 164
Bruch, Hilde, 82, 113
Bulimia, 7-27
   bingeing, 18-24
   closet nature of, 9
   life experiences that precede, 14
   obsession with thinness, 9
   one history of, 8-12
   Overeaters Anonymous, 10-11
   physical disorders of, 13-14
   physiological causes of, 14
   psychological impulsions to, 14-17
   self-worth, importance of, 15-17
   therapy for, 11-12, 17-18, 25-27
Bulimics
   characteristics of, 13-14
   life experiences inducing disease, 14
   therapy for, 11-12, 17-18, 25-27
   weight loss by, 168-69

California, University of, mouse study at, 168
Cincinnati, University of, Medical Center, 15
Clothing, significance of, 62-63, 68, 73-74, 103-06
   as behavior control, 103-04
   as definition of self, 103
   to project your self-identity, 105-06
   as test of whom you'd like to be, 104-05
Compulsivity, eating, 128-29, 130, 133, 135, 152, 153, 157
Control, bingeing and, 22-24, 25

Danowski, Thaddeus S., 168
Diet books, 1-2
Diets, 2
   failures of, 113
   physiological reasons for, 161-66, 168-69
   modifying for texture and temperature, 114
Discrimination in eating answering the need to eat, even without hunger, 139-40
   chocolate kiss exercise, 133-37
   "clean your plate" syndrome, getting over, 140-41
   eat what you want and still lose weight, 137
   inflexible work hours, getting around, 137-38
   nutrition vs. cravings, 142-43
   discover your own body's needs, 143
   others are eating, you're not hungry, 138-39
   restricted diets, coping with, 141
   you're hungry but nothing "hums," 139
Dublin, Louis I., 167
Duncan, Isadora, 75

Eating awareness. *See* Compulsivity, eating; Discrimination in eating; Eating behavior, nonjudgmental observation of; Emotional eating; Foods; Hunger; Self-regulatory mechanism of human body
Eating behavior, nonjudgmental observation of, 114-18
   chart, maintaining a, 117-18
   corrective feedback, 115-16
   inward focus not external stimuli, importance of, 116

Index

Eating Disorders, 82
Eating problems, 12
  difficulty of giving up your, 170-76
  getting over your, 178
Emotional eating, 58, 86, 118-19
Exercise (physical)
  and BMR, 168-69
  focus on specific body areas, 107
  yoga, 107
  not necessary for weight loss, 106
  set point theory, 108-09
  but valuable, 108, 109, 166
  should be done for desire, 74-76, 106-07
  trust body signals, 107-08, 109

Fantasies, directed or guided, 30, 35-57
  finding your guide, 39-40
    problems in communication, 41-43
  "If my fat had a voice," 46-52
    discussion afterward, 47-52
    preface to, 46
  nonguided association exercises, 52-57
    analyses of, 53-54, 54-57
    "Fat is . . . , thin is . . . ," 54
    "I need by fat to . . . ," 52
  "Part of the body you do not like," 43-46
    discussion afterward, 44-46
    preface to, 43
  relaxation as beginning, 36-38
  exercises for, 37-38
Fat
  men and, 2-3
  phobia, 16-17
  "power" of, 28
  used as excuse, 28, 30-31
  retrieving the power of, 28-35
    directed or guided fantasies, *see* Fantasies, directed or guided
    doing something with acquired knowledge, 33-34
    hypothetical case, 29-31, 32-33
    recognition of true problems, 29-33
  women and, 2, 3, 4-5
  See also Thin (thinness)
Fat cell theory, 163-64
Fat is a Feminist Issue, 93-94, 153
Fisher, Seymour, 91, 107
Flier, Jeffrey, 162-63
Fonda, Jane, 7
Food, as means of self-mothering, 155-56
Food, power of. *See* Power of food
Food denial, 74, 113
Foods
  "beckoning," 123-24
  eating awareness (fullness) exercise, 131-33
  eating awareness (tasting) exercise, 127-31
  food awareness exercise, 125-27
  guilt at eating forbidden, 135-36
  "humming," 123, 124
  no good or bad, wrong or right, except for you, 124, 129-30
  for various hungers, 121-23
Framingham, Massachusetts, (weight) study, 167-68

Gallwey, Timothy, 115
Gerrard, Don, 126-27, 129-30, 131
Getting Strong, 109

Health, Education and Welfare, U.S. Department of, 168-69
Helstein, Ivy, 86
"Humming" foods, 123, 124
Hunger
    areas where felt: gums and teeth, 123
    stomach, 121-22
    throat and mouth, 122
    tongue and lips, 123
    hunger awareness exercise, 120-21
    proper satisfactions for, recognizing, 121-23
        eating awareness (fullness) exercise, 131-33
        eating awareness (tasting) exercise, 127-31
        food awareness exercise, 125-27
    recognizing true, 118-20
Hypokalemia (low potassium levels, 13

Inner Game of Tennis, The, 115
It is okay to feel bad!, 156-57

Lance, Kathryn, 109
Lipoprotein lipase (LPL), 164
Losing weight, 160-78
    calorie reduction, 168-69
    finding *your* best weight, 160-61, 166, 169-70
    giving up your eating problem, difficulty of, 170-76
        fantasy personification of the part of you that holds on to your eating problem, 171-76
    now you are finally ready for, 176-78
    take it slowly!, 177-78
    permanent loss, achieving, 169-70
    readjusting concept of ideal weight, 166-68
    regaining lost weight, whys of, 161-66
        physical abnormalities of obesity, 161-65
        set point theory, 165-66

Mind, conscious and unconscious, 85
Mind Trips to Help You Lose Weight, 155
Minnesota, University of, Hospital, 14
Monroe, Marilyn, 83
Munter, Carol, 11, 89-90

"Never Too Thin to Feel Fat," 92
New York Times, 162
Newsweek, 167-68

One Bowl, 126-27, 129-30, 131
Orbach, Susie, 11, 12, 58, 61, 89-90, 93-94, 119, 153
Overeaters Anonymous (O.A.), 10-11

Pearson, Leonard and Lillian, 121
Power of food, 144-59
    exercise on, 145-46
        discussion of exercise, 146-47
    fantasy of, 147-52
    discussion of fantasy, 148-52
    placebo effect, 145, 159
    taking back its power from food, 149-52, 156-59
    transition period, difficulties of, 158
    "World without food" fantasy, 152-55

Index

discussion of, 153-55
Psychologist's Eat-Anything Diet, The, 121, 133

Relaxation training, 26
Rodin, Judith, 162
Rudnick, David, 14

Science 1982, 108-09
Self-esteem, 15-17, 26
Self-hypnosis to control weight, 1, 36-37
Self-image, 2-3, 9, 15-17, 26, 31, 50-51, 56-57, 60, 63, 67-69, 75-76, 77-80
Self-regulatory mechanism of human body, 111
    loss of balance in, 111-13
    dieting, fallacy of, 112-13
    poor child-rearing, 111-12
    nonjudgmental observation of eating behavior, 114-18
    chart, maintaining a, 117-18
    corrective feedback, 115-16
    inward focus, not external stimuli, importance of, 116
Set point theory, 108, 165-66
Sirlin, Joyce, 13

Therapy for bulimics, 11-12
    need for, 17

proper therapist, finding a, 17-18
treatment program, typical, 25-27
Thin (thinness), 58-80
    exercise fantasies on unconscious associations with, 61-80
    list of things put off until you get thin, 73-76
    personification of the part of you that won't let you get thin, 64-71
    visualization of self in a thin body, 71-73
    your distinctive qualities, 77-80
    physiological problems of attaining, 58-59
    in proper perspective, 176
    psychological realities of, 59-61 176
Thurman, Judith, 92
Triglycerides, 164

UCLA, eating disorders clinic at, 14

Walford, Roy L., 168
Women's needs, self-awareness of, 3-5
Wooley, Susan, 15